FOLKLORE, GENDER, AND AIDS IN MALAWI

GENDER AND CULTURAL STUDIES IN AFRICA AND THE DIASPORA

This book series spotlights the experiences of Africans on the continent and in its multiple and multilayered diasporas. Its objective is to make available publications that focus on people of African descent wherever they are located, targeting innovative research that derives questions, concepts, and theories from historical and contemporary experiences. The broad scope of the series includes gender scholarship as well as studies that engage with culture in all its complexities. From a variety of disciplinary, interdisciplinary, and transdisciplinary orientations, these studies engage current debates, address urgent questions, and open up new perspectives in African knowledge production.

PUBLISHED BY PALGRAVE:

Spatial Literacy: Contemporary Asante Women's Place-making
by Epifania Akosua Amoo-Adare

Folklore, Gender, and AIDS in Malawi: No Secret Under the Sun
by Anika Wilson

FOLKLORE, GENDER, AND AIDS IN MALAWI

NO SECRET UNDER THE SUN

Anika Wilson

palgrave
macmillan

FOLKLORE, GENDER, AND AIDS IN MALAWI

First published in 2013 by
PALGRAVE MACMILLAN®
in the United States—a division of St. Martin's Press LLC,
175 Fifth Avenue, New York, NY 10010.

Where this book is distributed in the UK, Europe and the rest of the world, this is by Palgrave Macmillan, a division of Macmillan Publishers Limited, registered in England, company number 785998, of Houndmills, Basingstoke, Hampshire RG21 6XS.

Palgrave Macmillan is the global academic imprint of the above companies and has companies and representatives throughout the world.

ISBN: 978–1–137–32244–9

Library of Congress Cataloging-in-Publication Data is available from the Library of Congress.

A catalogue record of the book is available from the British Library.

Design by Newgen Knowledge Works (P) Ltd., Chennai, India.

First edition: November 2013

To my mother Mary Jean Holland Wilson,
who bears all things, believes all things, hopes all things, and
endures all things for the love of her children

CONTENTS

ACKNOWLEDGMENTS

For those of you who took time to sit down with a stranger and share your words and your worlds, my sincere thanks go out to you. Without the gracious women and men I met in Malawi who welcomed me so warmly this book would not have been possible. For you and for those who assisted me in my research in a professional capacity (though I cannot call all your names here) this book draws together your voices of wisdom; it is also your book. For my dear friend and research assistant, Catherine Simkonda, I cannot imagine working with a kinder, more brilliant, more wonderful person. I thank God for you and for the opportunity to meet so many delightful people in so many different place in this endeavor. I have truly been blessed beyond my wildest imaginings.

This book was written in part during my years as a graduate student at the University of Pennsylvania Folklore and Folklife Program and also as junior faculty at the University of Wisconsin-Milwaukee. While there are many colleagues and friends whose support, advice, and feedback have contributed to my research and writing, I want especially to thank friends from my writing groups: Cindy Byrd, Linda Lee, Veronica Aplenc, Beth Spillman, Tami Williams, Ellen Amster, Shelleen Greene, and Nan Kim. I give special thanks to Dana Hercbergs who never fails to show enthusiasm and interest even the most nascent and half-formed ideas. I'm glad you're my friend. I want to express my gratitude to my advisors from the University of Pennsylvania, David Hufford, Dan Ben-Amos, and Lee Cassanelli who guided me through my doctoral work even when my program had been banished to a turret. You taught me to appreciate ways of knowing that others ignore. Susan Watkins made so much of my research possible by inviting me to be a graduate researcher in Malawi; your openness and enthusiasm about the work of your students changed the course of my life. Thank you!

The Malawi Diffusion and Ideational Change Project (funded by the NIH) helped to fund several research trips to Malawi and place me in a network of researchers and friends at home and abroad. There are so many of you who supported my work but I especially want to thank Pete Fleming (founder of Invest in Knowledge Initiative), Jenny Trinatapoli, Michelle Poulin, James Mwera, Joyce Anderson, and Moir Walita. A big thanks to Anne Mkandawire who hosted me for many months in Rumphi and Joyce Anderson who took me in in Mchinji and shared her stories with me.

Critical funding for this project also came from the University of Pennsylvania Fontaine Fellowship and Fontaine Dissertation Fellowship, a Foreign Language Area Studies Award, a Center for Africana Studies Dissertation Fellowship, and a UW-Milwaukee Graduate School Research Committee Award. Time for writing was further made possible through the Department of Africology Executive Committee at University of Wisconsin-Milwaukee, a University of Wisconsin System Center for Race and Ethnicity Faculty Diversity Research Award, and a UW-Milwaukee Center for Twenty-first Century Studies Fellowship.

My dear friends and colleagues in the Department of Africology have done so much to help me complete this project, both through feedback and the faith they had in me. Joyce Kirk and Winston Van Horne—thank you for your feedback on my proposal drafts. Sandra Jones, thanks for all the encouragement and always feeding me when I lack the proper snacks to make it through the day. Erin Winkler, you read and commented on the whole manuscript but also reminded me that I sometimes need to relax with 1990s hip hop and R&B.

So many friends have helped to support me emotionally and spiritually. I am so grateful to you my confidants and mentors. Cindy Groff Heiner, thanks for emergency editing services and all your prayers. To all my ladies of PGCF—I can't imagine what my life in Philadelphia would have been without my Bess Bayne, Monica Kurude, Mona Basta, Aileen Kim, Grace Lee, and Alexia Brown To my mentors and friends, Kevin Bauder, Sarah Mitchell, Dick Landis and Jean Landis—you helped me grow so much and to believe I had something to say that was worth sharing. We miss you Jean. I have been very blessed to complete this project in another wonderful city, Milwaukee, with the support of new and precious friends: Jill Owczarzak, Jen Mobley, Jessica Williams, Rob Ruzanic, Winson Chu, Karolina May, and Scott and Sharon Karstensen and many more.

Finally I want to thank my family, who refrained from teasing me for what seemed like an interminable period of studentship and instead supported me in myriad wonderful ways–Alake Wilson, Alona Williams, Markus Wilson, Malkum Wilson, Fredie Wilson, Fred Wilson and my mother, Mary Jean Holland Wilson, who after carrying me nine months was forced to labor again by reading an early draft of the book prospectus. I love you all.

CHAPTER 1

INTRODUCTION

In the late 1990s, the American media seemed to have some definite ideas about what was driving the AIDS epidemic in Central and Southern Africa to such startling proportions. Any casual observer of that time could hardly be blamed for thinking that high infection rates were due to some kind of "savage" culture wherein men raped babies as a cure for AIDS, sexuality was unregulated, condoms were shunned, and a continent of "failed" states was now doomed to physical annihilation and self-destruction. All the worst of old fashioned European "Dark Continent" imaginings were reanimated. In 1999, *Time Magazine* published an article entitled "An Epidemic of Rapes," which told the story of a woman in South Africa brutally raped and left in doubt of her HIV status. The article also spoke of a teenage girl who had been raped by her father. The author linked these rapes, as well as the many others being reported in South Africa at that time, to the fact that "many believe that raping a virgin will kill HIV" (Hawthorne, 1999). Some sources claimed that this was a common belief across "sub-Saharan Africa" that was fueling the high infection rates in the region while others have denied the existence of the practice altogether (Barnard, 2005; Jewkes et al., 2002).

When I first began conducting research in Malawi in 2003, such media messages, passively consumed, had an impact on the kinds of questions I asked. Indeed, though my first line of inquiry for my graduate research involved asking married women whether they had any concerns about HIV infection with regards to their husbands, I also asked them whether they had ever heard stories about men who raped virgins to be cured of AIDS. I wondered if there was any validity to these reports. Most people I spoke to either said they had not heard of this happening or they had heard of these things as "general stories" on the radio. However, there was one woman, Grace, I interviewed in 2006 in a village in Northern Malawi who spontaneously told us (myself and my research assistant) that she was connected to a story of a man who raped two little girls "for medicine." It was suspected that the two girls had been infected with HIV because of the assault. Grace tearfully told us that she was being accused of ultimately having given the girls HIV because that man was her boyfriend. It was believed that he had contracted HIV from Grace whose husband was said to have died of AIDS. The gossip about her was painful, especially stories about how her two frequently ailing children were beautiful because "AIDS kids are beautiful" and claims that the children would be dying soon also.

Grace seemed to embody the image of vulnerable, stigmatized, and violated woman as imagined by the media (Western and Malawian), local and international NGOs, and scholars. A stigmatized woman who's voice is silenced, unheard. There seemed to be something in the media stories I had heard back home. But looking back at the interview transcripts later I realized I had misunderstood Grace's story in several ways that would only become clear the longer I lived in Malawi. First, when Grace spoke of the man assaulting the young girls for "medicine", she did not explicitly reference HIV as the disease he hoped to be cured of. This is important because stories more commonly circulated are those about people who must sleep with a virgin (or someone with whom it is taboo to sleep—mother, sister, child, etc.) to activate medicine to increase wealth and good fortune. While this type of story, like those about the virgin cure, is also "sensational" it shifts the perspective from what is found interesting (or loathsome) to Western audiences to the concerns preoccupying Malawians. When hearing Grace's story, I first assumed that people must be seeking medicine for HIV, yet rumors and gossip in Malawi suggest some people want medicine for gaining money and material advancement or security. While AIDS looms large in the Western imaginings of "African" communities, even in the most epidemic stricken areas (specifically Southern Africa) people are contending with a multiplicity of priorities and concerns among which AIDS is only one.

My perspective shifted then—these stories about virgin cures were the ones "we" like to tell. What are the stories Malawian men and women want to tell, do tell? What narratives, whether mundane or outrageous, capture imaginations in Malawi? Informal folk narratives such as gossip, advice, rumor, and contemporary legends provide a unique lens through which to discern popular formulations of AIDS beliefs and marital conflict. This book presents Malawian narratives of love medicine, gossip about violent romantic rivalry, rumors of a mysterious and new sexually transmitted disease, common marital advice, and stories of rape accomplished through magic to gain insight into an era marked by social upheaval in Southern Africa. *Folklore, Gender, and AIDS in Malawi* begins with narratives of Malawian wives dealing with the risk of HIV infection introduced by their husbands and then opens up to present a broader set of narratives portraying contemporary marital struggles in a context of high AIDS prevalence, political transition, and economic insecurity. This book analyzes folk narratives to present local definitions of vulnerability and empowerment, risk perception and risk management, and knowledge and desire. Women and men desire more than just to avoid HIV. People also seek to maintain the relationships that imbue their lives with meaning, status, and a sense of belonging.

Women of Southern Africa have been portrayed by many scholars and journalists as victims of men in the AIDS epidemic. Whether as mothers and wives who are infected by roaming husbands or prostitutes forced by cruel economic circumstances to sell sex, a similar refrain of women's vulnerability has been sung for decades. This construction of women's vulnerability in Malawi has lead to the creation of many public health interventions targeted toward improving women's plights. However, often these well-intentioned programs instruct women to change their behavior without otherwise altering the social field in which they operate. Marriage is a particularly important institution in which many women operate thus the first part of the book (chapters 2 and 3) focuses on narratives specifically about marriage and marital conflict in a time of AIDS, while the last two chapters speak to a broader sense of gendered vulnerability to AIDS and women's position vis-à-vis men in sexual relationships. This book seeks not to deny women's vulnerability but to show how vulnerability is defined, navigated, and critiqued in informal, folkloric expression.

Informal narratives can produce knowledge that becomes the basis for action. The cautionary tales shared among peers and between elders and younger married couples are part of advice giving and therefore the narratives explicitly set the basis for action. Informal narratives also constitute disciplining discourses that prescribe behavior in subtle ways (Foucault, 1978). In other instances, gossip and rumor provide directed bases for action (Shibutani, 1966). In one village where I conducted interviews, the outrageous rumors about a man who was said to magically sleep with women at night caused the local women to rush for HIV testing. Even those who had experienced no characteristic dream or physical evidence associated with supernatural seduction made their way to a testing facility. There is nothing "idle" or trivial about gossip and other types of narratives that generate knowledge and action.

Ultimately, the narratives presented in this book display the intensely collective nature of problems and the correspondingly collective nature of problem solving, knowledge building, and social critique that occurs beneath the level of official interventions. While public health organizations around the world struggle to modify failing models and messages of individual behavior change, Malawians go about actively crafting responses to the epidemic in ways that are sensitive to the social basis of health and illness they encounter everyday. These narratives express both the strengths and limitations people experience in seeking to mitigate their risk of HIV infection and reimagine intimate relationships.

AIDS in Malawi

Malawi, like other countries in Southern Africa, is in the midst of an entrenched AIDS crisis. Three decades deep into the epidemic, Malawi's current HIV prevalence rate hovers at an estimated 10 percent among adults ages 15–49 (Department of Nutrition, HIV and AIDS, 2012: 2). The rate among that age group peaked at 16.4 in 1999 and then began declining. At the time of my initial interviews, men's prevalence rate was 10 percent and women's 13 percent (National Statistics Office [NSO], 2005: 230). HIV prevalence rates also vary according to whether one lives in a city or in a rural area. Urban women had a much higher HIV prevalence rate than rural woman (18 percent versus 13 percent), but the difference between urban and rural men was even more pronounced (16 percent and 9 percent, respectively), suggesting that whether in the city or on their farms, women have been more vulnerable to HIV infection than men (NSO, 2005: 17). Though an epidemic of these proportions has been decades in the making, the public health infrastructure has had little success in keeping pace with the need. Malawi, a small country located in Southeast Africa with a population of roughly 15 million, not only has one of the highest AIDS burdens, but it is one of the poorest nations in the world, a circumstance that adds to the difficulties in stemming the expansion of the disease.

In the mid-1980s, Malawi's government instituted strategies for battling the spreading epidemic. Since the drafting of the first strategic plan, HIV/AIDS programs have been primarily geared toward activities of testing, creating "awareness," preventing mother-to-child-transmission (PMTCT), and promoting behavior change (Department of Nutrition, HIV and AIDS, 2005). With scarce resources and a weak public health infrastructure, the government provided relatively little in the way of treatment. According to Malawi's own Ministry of Health, of more than 20,000 healthcare posts, 33 percent are vacant, a total of 64 percent of nursing positions had not been filled, and Malawian healthcare facilities retains only one-sixth of the number of recommended doctors (Harries et al., 2006: 1070). It was only in 2005 that the government began dispensing, free of charge, anti-retroviral drugs (ARVs), which lengthen the lives of AIDS sufferers; a decade earlier these drugs had transformed AIDS into a chronic disease in rich nations (Palella et al., 1998).

To a great extent, the government's current provision of ARVs has been made possible by external donors, most notably the Global Fund to fight AIDS, Tuberculosis, and Malaria (Harries, 2006: 1071). The newly democratic government, with its assets of democracy and "good governance," was able to attract substantial donor funds to address the problem that Malawi's own underfunded public health system could not. By the late 1990s, one researcher estimated that at least seventy-three nongovernmental organizations (NGOs), both local and international, were dealing with AIDS in Malawi, the largest contributors being UNAIDS, USAID, UNDP, UNICEF, Action-Aid, and the British governmental aid agency DFID. By 2009, approximately 200,000 Malawians were receiving free ARVs (HIV and AIDS Monitoring and Evaluation Report, 2008–2009).

Despite the government's coordination of ARV distribution, external donors and NGOs appear to have considerable influence in the distribution and usage of AIDS funds. The extension of influence of international nongovernmental sector and multilateral organizations on policies and practices in resource poor nations like Malawi has been described as transnational governmentality (Englund, 2006). Since the 1970s, NGOs have been viewed as a preferred route through which international donor funds flow, particularly in sub-Saharan African nations whose governments have been branded as corrupt, inefficient, and not accountable to citizens; by contrast, NGOs are perceived as stable, honest, and participatory entities (Morfit, 2011: 2). Morfit suggests that NGOs' special focus on "AIDS in Africa" draws funds and attention away from equally pressing developmental issues and distorts the missions of various agencies. The proliferation of AIDS-related organizations or affiliations has been described by some Malawians as constituting an "AIDS Industry" wherein employees or volunteers receive benefits of pay, travel, status, and other various amenities as they "sensitize" the "masses" to the dangers of HIV/AIDS (Wilson, 2008). Messages routed through the "AIDS Industry" are sometimes welcomed and sometimes met with ambivalence. These messages are supplemented by thriving informal information dissemination and discussion that I explored in my fieldwork and narrative collection.

Fieldwork

The topics I chose to research emerged from preliminary fieldwork in Malawi during the summers of 2004 and 2005 in conjunction with my participation in the Malawi Diffusion and Ideational Change Project (MDICP). [1] The MDICP is a longitudinal survey project that solicits data on the impact of social networks in the dissemination of health information and behavior change. The project has a qualitative component, a journal project in which Malawians, trained to work as interviewers for MDICP, write down everyday conversations about AIDS they overhear or take part in. During my assignments as a graduate research assistant, one of my responsibilities was thematically coding such reports.[2]

While coding, I realized that these everyday conversations are a major means by which health information is imparted, debated, and reinterpreted; the stories being told about HIV and AIDS were stories about infidelity, sick neighbors and their symptoms, rich men enticing young girls with money, women fighting over men, scandals of men and women caught in the act of "Illicit" sexual intercourse, concern about the youth and the "nowadays disease," discussions of biomedical treatment of AIDS versus treatment by traditional healers (*sing'anga*), men and women fretting over how to choose a sex partner or spouse, and controversies over the efficacy and morality of condom use. People debated the usefulness of testing and speculated about the merit of revealing one's HIV status. There were complaints about local health-care workers and wasteful government spending. Through these stories, I was drawn to study rumor, gossip, and conspiracy theory as processes of health belief formation. As people try to make sense of the magnitude and impact of AIDS on the nation and in their communities, they come together to actively seek and constitute knowledge.

The strength of the ethnographic journals is that they give a glimpse into natural conversation and the ways in which themes of narratives flow one into another, displaying cognitive links. My initial forays into villages of Northern Malawi helped me in shaping a course of inquiry that included both guided interviews and an expanded journal project I designed to focus specifically on marital conflict and women's prevention strategies.

In addition to collecting journals, I conducted interviews with the aid of a research assistant, Catherine Simkonda. Our aim was to engage in conversation with women who had been married within a particular village so that we might hear multiple versions of a story to better grasp the distribution of information and its varying interpretations. After choosing the particular village, we interviewed women based on their marital status and willingness to be interviewed; some respondents were found by just approaching homes and asking to speak to married women there. After those interviews, we asked for referrals to other women within that compound, creating a snowball sample. Sometimes we moved on from one compound to another without a reference when there seemed to be no more married women available or when practical concerns arose; for example, we once moved on to a new compound because it was too difficult for Catherine Simkonda to walk up the hill in the previous village as her pregnancy progressed.[3] We interviewed in five compounds of a single village between January 2005 and May 2006.

With the help of a research assistant and interpreter, I conducted my interviews with married women in one particular village, Chikuwala, near Phukwa's provincial trading center. Chikuwala is situated below a tarmac that connects to Mzuzu (the city of the north) in one direction and to the nexus of Malawi, Tanzania, and Zambia in the other. Though not a hub for governmental administration, Phukwa (a pseudonym for the small trading center; the word means "to desire") is an educational center having both men's and women's technical schools as well as a nationally renowned secondary school. Down the road from the polytechnic schools is the Phukwa market, where many of my informants purchased the groceries they did not produce themselves and sold mangoes and stalks of sugar cane. Phukwa boasted a bar and a resthouse which loomed large in the imagination of wives in Chikuwala, becoming a synecdochic referent for prostitution and men's mobility and adultery.

We interviewed 60 women and a subset of 15 were chosen to be visited a second and third time. With each visit, we were updated on developments in relevant narratives. This method is similar to the social anthropology "extended-case study method" that developed in the 1950s and 1960s in studies of witchcraft, urbanization, and modernization. Put simply, this method follows the conflicts of particular persons as they develop over time and is particularly suited to the study of conflict and the processes that bring about change. Englund states,"The actual relations of Tom, Dick and Harry' could themselves generate processes that circumvented or modified general principles—processes that were not, however, utterly devoid of logic" (Englund, 2002a: 28–29).[4] The extended case method is useful because situations are not discrete and conflicts of everyday life are ongoing. The decisions and events of today, though dramatic, can be overturned tomorrow. The same can be said of the narratives that relate to events. As an interested public keeps tabs on a particular conflict, the observations and judgments of today can be replaced by new information.

During subsequent research trips (2008 and 2010) I interviewed people in the Central and Southern regions of Malawi on broadly circulating rumors featured in chapters 4 and 5. Media reports, casual conversations scribbled in field notes, and journal writings alerted me to rumors about a supposedly new sexually transmitted disease and to rumors about *mgoneko* sexual assault magic. These sources served as a jumping off point for further inquiries that I pursued through interviews in Zomba (Southern Malawi), Mchinji (Central Malawi), and Rumphi (Northern Malawi). Not only did newspaper reports serve as important site for the reporting of rumor and urban legends, they are a subject of inquiry in the last chapter as informal discourses move between word of mouth and printed circulation. The final chapter of this book deals most with media, which are conduits of urban legend in the Malawian context (and indeed many places around the world).

My journal project, modeled on the MDICP journal project, was initiated in July 2005. In the summer of 2005, I recruited five Rumphi residents to write down conversations they heard in the course of the day. Part of my motivation for this comes from the difficulty of entering gossip networks as an outsider. Working with locals becomes an important means for accessing information that flows in intimate networks. Merry describes this dilemma for participant-observers, writing, "I was able to trace the flow of information circulating around the neighborhood, but I had little access to those intimate moments when close friends talk about a third friend. I expect this is true for much ethnography on gossip. Gossip may be a phenomenon that must rely heavily on reports of participants rather than those of observers" (Merry, 1984: 273). The journal project was an answer to that dilemma. Although a journal project already existed that had collected over 500 reports, most of these reports were coming out of the predominantly matrilineal, Muslim Southern district of Balaka; there was little coverage of Northern districts.

In July 2005, I recruited two women and three men in Rumphi ranging from ages 17 to 28 who had all completed high school and were fluent in English. The men and women were recruited during the hiring process for the Malawi Religion Project (MRP), a sister project to MDICP in which data collection took place during the summer of 2005. I worked as a graduate student assistant for MRP and those who hired interviewers and trained them referred five of the trainees to me to work as journalers. Both male and female journalers[5] were included to provide insights into the conversations that take place between men and men; men and women; and women and women. All were instructed to attend to gossip, rumor or scandal relating to topics of interest that included stories about marital conflicts, HIV/AIDS, and witchcraft. I refer to these men and women as "journalers." The journalers were told that they could engage in normal conversations but should not act as formal interviewers. They should write a record of the conversation on the same night it took place. The journals were to be written in such a way as to reflect the back-and-forth dynamic of conversation and were to be written as close to verbatim as possible.

While I encouraged the journalers to be listeners more than speakers or initiators of conversations, I found upon reviewing their writing that for journalers to initiate conversations was a natural part of interaction and that what it means to initiate a conversation is not simple to discern. I discovered that a relevant conversation[6] could be initiated by a question or an observation that sparks a conversation. Some journalers, especially Simon Nyirenda who had no other employment at the time would spend time visiting the market and other public places in order to listen and insert his questions into a conversations already taking place. The effect of this was that the speakers sometimes discussed aspects of the topic they may not have otherwise mentioned. Yet the question and answer exchange is a part of the way in which people conversed. If Simon had been mute, this may have seemed strange and shown a lack of interest on his part. By contrast, several times the journaler Hastings Mkandawire came upon a situation and asked a question that sparked an discussion that he could not have known would lead to the kinds of conversations in which I was interested. When he saw a burnt house near the home he was visiting he asked what happened and was told a story of a jealous wife burning the home of her rival. In another instance, when Hastings, a craftsman and a farmer, went to buy fertilizer, he began chatting with one of his clients, Mrs.Mwandira, a married woman in her 30s. As the two talked a young woman named Beatrice came to her to borrow money. Hastings had questions about the woman when she walked away.

Hastings: Are you related to this beautiful lady?

Mrs.Mwandira: Oh yes she is a relative of my husband she is the daughter of my husband's aunt.

Hastings: She is beautiful I tell you I have liked her who can do the work for me? *(Mrs. Mwandira laughed before giving me a question.)*

Mrs.Mwandira: What work do you want somebody to do for you?

Hastings: I have loved her, but I am afraid to propose her direct, and instead I need somebody to do the work on my behalf—somebody like you.

(Mrs. Mwandira laughed and asked me if I was alone) I am not alone, I am married but I wanted to have her too. I feel like there can't be a problem to have her in my house. *(In fact I was not all serious playing that game but I really pretended serious this was one way of passing hours away while waiting along cue[sic] to be going.)*

Mrs.Mwandira: Do you know Rabson Kamanga of Mphombo Village?

Hastings: Oh yes, I know that boy what about him, are they going out together or do you want to tell me that Rabson wants to marry her?

Mrs.Mwandira: Mr. Craftsman, do you stay in Mphokwa? Rabson once married that lady—he was the sixth husband since she started changing husbands.

Hastings: I heard that Rabson has married but I didn't know that he married this beautiful lady—so you mean she is already divorced.

Mrs.Mwandira: Mister, beauty has nothing to do in life and love, my reaction is [that she is] really beautiful but her behavior is not beautiful. As I am talking Beatrice is pregnant and she is HIV positive so if you are ready to take care of the double troubles then I will do that work on your behalf.

Hastings: You may know about the pregnancy, but it's difficult for you to know that the lady is HIV positive, unless you know her hospital report after an HIV test.

Mrs.Mwandira: We know some of the husbands whom she was married to—they were carrying all signs of being HIV positive.

(Beatrice came close to where [we] were. I don't know what was she to do this time we stopped talking and started other stories. I even stopped admiring the woman for what I got clearly showed that the lady was just beautiful out ward looking but the inside was not okey.) (Mkandawire research journal, January 2008)

In the excerpt above, Hastings comment clearly sparked the part of the conversation that eventually lead Mrs. Mwandira to disclose the scandalous history of Beatrice. However, he could not have known that the woman's reputation was tarnished when he began his playful banter. Hastings continued to prompt Mrs. Mwandira to disclose more information with follow-up questions and the proffering of his opinions. Yet even his promptings were not such that they were designed to elicit a particular kind of history. They were not the kind of direct questioning that I sought to avoid such as "Do you know of any women or men who are reputed to have contracted AIDS through their sexual activities?" or "Have you heard of any marital conflicts occurring recently?" Instead the questions and observations made by Hastings and the other journalers arose from the social context of the moment.

I suggested the journalers write their entries in the form of a play, focusing primarily on displaying the dialogue. Some followed this instruction better than others. Though the journals were written primarily in English, great latitude was given for the journaler to write out long phrases in chiTumbuka[7] and then translate on the same page. The original instruction was for journalers to write out proverbial statements or axiomatic phrases in chiTumbuka and include a translation. Later, I could see that some journalers found it useful to write out other types of phrases in the original language for the sake of recall. The innovation was accepted as a normal part of the journal project.

The journals were written in standard 80-page exercise books (20 × 14.5 cm) designed for use by Malawian primary and secondary school students. Journalers were compensated about $20.00 for each booklet and could complete two per month. The limit was set to decrease the temptation of fabricating stories. Of course, there are no guarantees that journalers, or I daresay any informant, is completely honest, but the limit was a hedge against dishonesty. The topics I was interested in were popular topics for discussion, and so I assumed there would be no lack of real discourse for the journalers to record. Furthermore, journalers were asked to give details about the context of the conversation, the relationships among those involved in the discussion, and a description of all those present.

Anyone who has ever written field notes knows that it is quite easy to write indefinitely on one event, one moment. Journalers were permitted to write freely and to update stories they had written down before if they heard a new conversation on the same topic; thus there was plenty of material to keep journalers busy without the need for falsification. The use of local journalers to collect information, like all methods, has limitations. The high monetary compensation (compared with what most Malawians earned), as mentioned above, could act as an incentive for journalers to fill booklets with fake stories or rambling narratives. However, issues of trust and reliability are present in all research that relies upon the witness of informants. I had some assistance in gauging not only the factuality of reports but also the plausibility of the stories therein. Both my research assistant and a typist gave comments on the relative quality and plausibility of the journalers from a cultural insiders' perspective. Their input aided me in ranking the work of the journalers relative to one another so that I could decide whose work needed to be eyed with greatest skepticism and whose work was the most reliable.

In addition, I hoped to find overlap in the stories discussed by journalers who lived in the same region. Yet I discovered only one instance in which two journalists, as well as an interview respondent, all discussed a particular woman, Agnes. From the journaler Hastings Mkandawire we learn that Agnes once lived in Mzuzu but after an unspecified scandal involving a man she returned HIV positive to her grandmother's home to live. Hastings notes two separate conversations about Agnes, one in which people discussed a fight she had with her grandmother and her failed marriage and another conversation in which people discussed her HIV positive status, her use of ARVs, and her marital prospects. Another journaler, Tawonga Msowoya, chronicled a conversation she had with Agnes in which she sought to offer comfort to Agnes when she was despairing about her health. And finally, in the village where I interviewed married women, located near the village of Hastings and Tawonga, we asked women if they had ever heard of anyone who sought to spread the HIV virus on purpose. One of the women told us that Agnes was such a person who "accepts every man that goes for her and they do everything they want with her." Later our respondent insisted Agnes "has killed a lot of people. Some even cry telling her that she has killed them." The multiple references to Agnes points to a real circulation of information about her rather than a fabrication of incidents by each journaler. This overlap helps to lend credence to the honesty of the journalers more generally. However, the multiple reports of Agnes' story by several journalers was the exception rather than the rule. This leads to the tentative conclusion that within the same geographical space[8] multiple social networks co-exist among which people are not necessarily preoccupied with discussing the same subjects. What was recurrent was not particular stories about particular people but rather types of stories, genres.

The other drawback of using journals is that they are not verbatim records. This means that they are more suited for capturing meanings and sequences of conversational transitions than they are suited for deeper structural linguistic analysis. In this they are quite similar to an ethnographer's field notes which also fail to capture exact language. However, the impressions of reality jotted down by the journalists are full of descriptive detail, debate, and local wisdom which in its cumulative weight across journalers and over time (some journalers wrote for about a year and others for multiple years) is substantial.

During my stay in Malawi between November 2005 and June 2006, I met the journalers to collect the journals once a month. At the end of my 2005–2006 fieldwork project I had gathered over one hundred journals. Since then many more have been written and typed. While the original guidelines I gave were broad and covered a range of conflicts and scandals that may have arisen, as my focus narrowed and my funds depleted it was necessary to limit the number of documents which could be typed. Throughout this document all references to proper names or people and places have been replaced with exception of major marketplaces, townships, districts, NGOs, and public figures (e.g., a reference to Malawi's President remains specific). Between 2005 to date, I have continued to collect journals but on a more sporadic basis; I have narrowed my collection to one or two journalers at a time.

Because Hastings Mkandawire tends to express himself in a clear, detailed manner and have a wide and varied social network, his contributions have been particularly helpful. Mkandawire (born in the late 1970s) is my longest running journaler. He began working with me in 2005 and continues to this time (December 2012). Mkandawire first aspired to be a schoolteacher but was not able to get a spot in the University of Malawi after finishing secondary school. When that scheme failed, he turned to craft school that he completed with distinction. He set up shop alongside the tarmac not far from a trading center, secondary school, and technical schools. Alongside his sales of crafts he relies on other sources of financial gain including agriculture and involvement in research projects (like mine).

In a 2012 interview conducted by Catherine Simkonda, Mkandawire says that after the many years of writing journals writing is "now in his blood." To him the experience of talking to people is "like going for more education." His tried and true method (according to his own report) is to crack a joke to which someone will often reply that the thing he has described really happened. From this a person will describe a long story. Mkandawire then acts as if he does not know such things happen to encourage the storyteller to elaborate. On occasion he will sometimes buy a drink for the person so the conversation will continue longer. He makes the point of always being alert to new gossip or rumors and writes them as soon as possible, taking advantage of his proclivity to go to bed after others.

He feels that he is a good journaler because he interacts with a wide cross-section of people well and often; owing to his business dealings and his role as an unofficial role as counselor in his church and favor granter in his community, his acquaintance is wide. When asked why he elected to include stories about his own marital strife, he said he felt that he tells his stories so that others could benefit and also because he saw no reason why he should not also "sell" his own story. He muddled through without acquiring a second wife to join his first wife because he was concerned creating a polygamous family like the one he was raised in wherein he suffered from a lack of resources and also from his father's drinking problem. He has his own family with a wife, their four children, and a fifth child from outside the marriage.

Marriage in Malawi

A major portion of my field research took place among the Tumbuka of Northern Malawi between 2005 and 2006. It is in this context that

I studied women's marital strategies for preventing AIDS infection. Malawi is divided into three large administrative districts that correspond roughly to ethnic groupings. The district of Rumphi sits in the Northern region, which has been politically and economically marginalized since independence in 1964, stagnating industrial development and political representation (Friedson, 1996: 52; Vail and White, 1989). Most Tumbuka are subsistence farmers, living on extended-family compounds and cultivating a plot of land to support the family. Crop surpluses are often used to buy soap, salt, sugar for tea, and to pay school fees (Friedson, 1996: 53).

Although the Northern region is politically and economically marginalized in comparison to the other regions, Rumphi has high average educational attainment in contrast to districts in the Central and Southern regions. In a survey, 93 percent of Tumbuka men responded that they could read and write, while only 51 percent of the Yao and Chewa men could. Of Tumbuka women 70 percent were literate, whereas among Yao women only 12 percent were literate (Poulin, 2007: 97f). The greater emphasis on education relative to other regions is likely due to the legacy of missionaries from the Free Church of Scotland who came to the area in the late nineteenth century. Another legacy of the missions in the North is a high concentration of Presbyterians compared to the Central region, where Catholicism dominates, and Southern Malawi, where Islam has a major following.

In my research site, the village of Chikuwala,[9] as in many villages in Northern Malawi, the economy is dominated by the production and sale of tobacco. A labor-intensive enterprise with unpredictable returns, growing tobacco often involves the hiring of additional laborers outside the household, the shifting of adolescent plants from the *dambo* (fertile wetlands) nurseries to the fields, and the liberal use of costly fertilizer. The division of labor between men and women is striking. In addition to cultivating cash and subsistence crops, other economic activities in Rumphi included the ownership of small tack shops,[10] teaching, trade, and selling crafts (Takane, 2006). Most non-agricultural cash-generating activities are dominated by men who are more mobile than women, leaving women dependent on men for provision of cash for school fees and other such necessities (Kerr, 2005a).

Marriage among the Tumbuka is patrilineal and virilocal. Generally speaking, women are closely tied to the domestic sphere of their affinal kin by a multitude of productive and reproductive responsibilities. While men and women both work in agricultural production, women additionally keep the home through daily cleaning and periodic smearing.[11] The village where I carried out my research was composed of several compounds where close patrikin live in clustered houses of mud wall or mud brick and thatch. Here the women cooked—sometimes for in-laws or the whole compound—cared for the children, took care of ailing family members, and spent hours fetching firewood and drawing water. On average women in Malawi work a twelve-hour work day, whereas men work from four to six hours per day (Schatz, 2002: 50). Quoted in Schatz (2002), Mbilizi states that "The fact that women work exceedingly hard for survival has made them the most vulnerable group" (Mbilizi, 1997; Schatz, 2002). And while women hear the many public health warnings about AIDS, it is not necessarily at the top of their daily concerns; women must also contend with child care, care of the sick, responsibilities to relatives at home and in their marital village, agricultural work, and more. However, marriage practices (and the gendered roles associated with them) in Malawi are far more ambiguous, flexible, and subject to transformations than the labels "matrilineal" and "patrilineal" systems suggest. Similarly the ethnic or "tribal designations" used to describe Malawians (and other Africans) creates a false impression of distinctiveness in language, custom, and interaction than is reflected by the reality (Kaspin, 1995; Posner, 2004). Trends in marriage practices among various communities in Malawi were profoundly affected by the trajectories of mobile populations, the slave trade, religious influences from Europe (Christianity) and the East coast (Islam), transformations of economic structures, and colonial policies in the ninteenth and twentieth centuries.

Before the ninteenth century, Tumbuka peoples of Northern Malawi tended toward matrilinearity with descent traced through mother's side and land inherited and managed through the mother. When married a couple would generally live uxorilocally, that is, with the wife's family. A groom would provide bride service to his in-laws. With the incursion and subsequent dominance of the Ngoni from Natal in South Africa in the late ninteenth century marriage practices of the Tumbuka shifted. The Ngoni (who broke away from the Zulu) imposed patrilineal descent and the payment of lobola as they intermarried with the conquered Tumbuka. Gradually matrilineal practices gave way to more patrilineal ones, though some aspects of matrilineality abide (Kerr, 2005a, 2005b; Young, 1931). Further encouraging increasingly patrilineal patterns in Malawi (in the Northern regions as well as in the rest of the country) were the British colonial administrators and Christian missionaries who saw patrilineality as closer to their own vision of idealized family structure. This family structure included a male head and a nuclear family organization as the unit of administration, taxation, and labor.

Similar processes were underway in Southern and Central Malawi. In the these regions where a large contingent of the matrilineal, uxorilocal Chewa, Yao, Nyanja now reside, changes in marital practices were also spurred by the slave trade of the ninteenth century, by colonial policies, such as hut taxes, and religious influences. Coming from Mozambique the Yao traded slaves in the Shire valley of Southern Malawi, many of whom were women. Men in places where matrilineal, uxorilocal marriages predominated and who did not want to live under the authority of in-laws or perform bride service, saw taking slave brides as an alternative. Otherwise they came as "strangers" to the villages of their wives. At the same time, their traditions already included options for chiefs and some ordinary men to live outside of their wives' villages or bring their wives back to their village. Among the Yao and Nyanja men could also marry a cross cousin so as to stay in their area of their kin group (Kachapila, 2006; Phiri, 1983; Power, 1995). The imposition of taxes and the mandate for people in certain regions to work on colonial estates spurred men to leave their homes for wage labor opportunities, creating new patterns of residence (e.g., urbanization, oscillating migration, neo-local residence upon marriage), as well as modification to the gendered division of labor. Women became increasingly responsible for a wider range of agricultural activities and reliant upon male wage labor for agricultural inputs (such as fertilizer). Some women who could not rely of remittances from males came to rely upon *ganyu* labor practices, a kind of sharecropping or "piece work" for farmers with larger land holdings (Kerr, 2005b).

Marriage practices were further impacted by the expansion of mission Christianity in Malawi (especially Presbyterianism and Catholicism) with its emphasis of male-headed nuclear families and denigration of polygamy (Phiri, 1983: 268). Some have linked the spread of Christianity in Malawi—in conjunction with the growth of wage labor, urbanization, labor migration—with increasing individualization in choice of marital partner and increasing atomization of the family away from more extended family units such as the *mbumba*, "the consanguineously related women reckoning back to a founding ancestress" (Power, 1995: 81). The *mbumba* (in matrilineal Central and Southern Malawian groups) is headed by a senior male on the woman's side and functions to structure social life in terms of mediating disputes, marriages, and land allocation. Processes of atomization and individualization thus also pose challenges to gerontocratic authority as decisions about marriage are also linked to control of labor and intergenerational exchange.

According to Clark et al. (2009) adolescents and young adults now have greater autonomy in choosing their mates than ever before, but choices are complicated by the AIDS epidemic. Some of my informants who were elders complained that AIDS has come for their children because the youth do not listen to them with respect to advice about marriage and sex. Heterosexual relationships, while not confined to marriage, have been described as "under the shadow of marriage;" Anne Griffiths has shown in her study of procreative relationships in Botswana, that even when a couple is not married the logics of marriage (and by extension the gendered inequalities thereof) impact the claims men and women make on each other (1997). Indeed, Clark et al. have shown that anticipation of marriage can effect whether and how unmarried adolescents engage in sexual relationships (2009). The last chapters of this volume draw upon some narratives in which the key figures are not married; yet the sex-related conflicts I describe arise from the disjunctures perceived between the idealized role of a woman as wife/mother in the village and the fear of mobile, unattached, and sexually voracious women (chapter 4). In the next chapter, marriage is sometimes explicitly referenced and other times it is the anticipation of sexual relationships ordered by a gendered hierarchy enshrined in marriage (law and practice) that causes concern.

What is it that people expect and hope for in their marriages? When asked what the most desirable qualities were in a potential spouse many young men and women across Malawi named being HIV negative, educated, and skilled at cooking and cleaning as high on the list. Also high on the list was faithfulness. About 30 percent of men and women named fidelity as important characteristics in a future spouse (Clark et al., 2009).

Despite increasing atomization in marriages wherein the conjugal pair becomes the primary locus of economic and social reproduction, my research shows the continued salience of larger family structures in ordering these relations. To understand Malawian women's responses to the AIDS crisis, we must first understand their embeddedness in multiple relations of responsibility. One major complaint of women in Malawi is that while they may adhere to the ABCs (the acronym for the three-pronged public health campaign for AIDS prevention message, well known in sub-Saharan Africa: *A*bstain, *B*e Faithful, Use *C*ondoms. See Sinding (2005)), they do not trust their husbands to do so. Yet women are bound (and/or inclined) by expectations of marriage to consent to sex with husbands even when they feel endangered by them. Few wives are in the position to insist on the use of condoms within their marriage (Caldwell et al., 1997; Lane, 2004; Mutongi, 1999; Ulin, 1992; Whyte, 1997). This may explain why so many strategies I learned about involve trying to change the behavior of the "other." There were two main types of "other" that women's strategies targeted: husbands and the extramarital partners of their husbands. Many of these strategies discussed in chapters 2 and 3 may be seen more generally as strategies for ensuring the fidelity of a spouse, but in these times of the "nowadays disease," (a local name for AIDS) ensuring fidelity takes on a new level of urgency such that even some extreme actions may be tacitly endorsed by sympathetic community members. Indeed, for a woman to influence her husband or his other significant other, her ability to garner community support is key. It is through various community members that useful knowledge is passed that helps to navigate complex relationships in dangerous times.

By contrast, sources of information about AIDS, such as the government and public health education interventions spearheaded by NGOs, represent official orthodoxies. These official sources provide vital basic information about HIV/AIDS, but this information has its limitations of usefulness and trustworthiness.

AIDS Messages and Interventions: Government, Media, and NGOs

HIV/AIDS is known by many names in Malawi. It is called *edzi* (playing off the pronunciation of the English acronym), *nthenda yatsopano* (the new disease), *kachirombo* ("little animal/beast"), among others. The government is a dominant organizational referent for HIV/AIDS in Malawi; one popular name for AIDS is *Matenda a Boma*, translated "government disease" (Lwanda, 2005; Peters, Kambewa, and Walker, 2010). The nature of the perceived connection is varied. For some the connection comes from first hearing of AIDS from government announcements. During research conducted in 2004, we asked village headmen and traditional healers in rural Rumphi District when they first remember hearing about AIDS.

The following conversation with a traditional healer typifies the responses offered:

> I asked when he first began to notice AIDS and what he, as a healer, does about it. He [said he] started hearing about HIV/AIDS in the'80s and '90s. He saw this [AIDS] in action starting 2001 to 2004 after seeing the sick people...He added that he was hearing about AIDS through the radio. We asked if he could remember what they were saying [on the radio].
>
> He said he was hearing from the people that there was AIDS, a disease that cannot be cured by traditional healers or doctors. They gave instructions—no local injections in the villages, take care of yourself. When going to healer carry your own razor blades. (Wilson field notes, July 16, 2004)

Msiska, a young healer and farmer, gained his initial knowledge of AIDS, like many others, not through firsthand experience but through warnings made on the radio, at government hospitals, or by word of mouth. Before the media was liberalized in 1994, the Malawi Broadcasting Corporation (MBC) was the only radio station in operation. It was also owned and tightly controlled by the then-autocratic, single-party national government (Chirambo, 2002: 112; Englund, 2002b: 22). The 1990s saw the high HIV prevalence of the 1980s converted into cases of full-blown AIDS and rapid deaths as people began to shrink to skeletal proportions, exhibiting the signs and symptoms described by government health officials. The messages of the government were thus the words of prophets.

In the passage below a man explains to the rumor journaler signs of AIDS and the reason that people should already be aware of these symptoms.

> "[It's] bad, this disease is killing those who are deaf enough from the daily messages from this radio (There was a radio near where he sat)...warning them that the disease is dangerous and has no medicine. What kind of disease has no medicine? In the past there were other dangerous disease[s] like *Chitayo* but [we] had medicine and the other but not this one."

And I asked..."[what do] these people think of this disease then?"

> He said "people think that because it is a global crisis and has world widely spread then it's indeed a disease which the bible has written about *Kaliwonde-wonde*."[12]
>
> And I said "What do they do, if [anything] at all, considering that partners they go for might have infected of this disease?"
>
> He said, "I believe some people are clever when noticing that his/her partner has started showing signs of what kinds of what the radio says that becoming...thinner and thinner, coughing persistently and hairs becoming scraggly and soft. The clever partners leaves or divorces the partner or the spouse no matter how good and powerful she was or he was to avoiding contracting the disease." (Bato, MDICP research journal, May 2002)

Here the media, radio specifically, is featured as an important source of knowledge about AIDS that can be used in devising strategies for avoiding the disease. The government, by its association with the media also gains further legitimacy through the assertion of the truth of HIV/AIDS messages. Malawi's first radio station, MBC, served as a mouthpiece for single-party government propaganda. Under the democratic dispensation, however, independent radio stations have sprung up.

Yet MBC remains dominant and the memory of the old authoritarian use of the media has not yet faded and some are suspicious that the media and the government conceal and distort information or subvert values held by the public. The public often suspects that the government is a censor or final approver of any information broadcast. For instance, conversations found in the rumor journals are full of complaints that the government is encouraging people to use Chishango brand condoms and thus encouraging extramarital sex and the spread of AIDS. Others complain that they are hawking defective goods, as the wife of one of the journalers asserts in the passage below:

> "The radio announces another type of Chishango condom which the government has yet just established. Why is the government recommending the new-fashioned type every day? It means the old ones have faults. Shouldn't they stop wasting money on this but rather make us aware of AIDS?" (Bato, MDICP research journal, April 2002)

Chishango is a brand of condoms distributed by Population Services International (PSI), a US-based NGO, and yet in many conversations it is the Malawian government that remains the focus of condom-related criticisms.

> "This is so because when you open the radio you hear that there is AIDS, when you attend a meeting you hear that there is AIDS, when you go to the church you hear that there is AIDS. It is heard everywhere that there is AIDS and because of that the guys are afraid of going for girls because they are afraid of catching AIDS. It is heard everywhere that there is AIDS and if there is a place where it is not common to hear of AIDS is at the funeral. I only heard once at a certain funeral at Kalonga where the village headman announced that the dead person had died of "*matenda a boma*." (Geladi, MDICP research journal, February 2003)

Along with the government, NGOs like PSI are responsible for a great deal of content in radio and newspaper. When in 2005 I interviewed media representatives (radio executives and programmers from MBC and Radio Maria, as well as a feature writer from Malawi's *The Nation* newspaper) aspects of the linkages between the media, NGOs and the government were made apparent. The media regularly feature representatives of the government, NGOs, and religious organizations to provide expert commentary on social, political, economic, and health issues. Highly educated Malawians often move between these institutions. A programmer at MBC, Willy Man'ganda, said that he helped to incorporate health-related (including AIDS-related) features in the programming. Before working for MBC, he was a public health officer for Malawi's Ministry of Health and a District AIDS Commission Coordinator in Machinga. He also worked for the NGO Banja La Mtsogolo, a family planning and sexual health organization associated with British/Welsh Maria Stopes International, operating in Malawi. When I met Mang'anda, he had just been made head of a new project for "mainstreaming" AIDS into MBC operations and programming, meaning that AIDS issues would be incorporated in various programs but also would be made part of the organizational functions of MBC more generally. The funding for this project was supplied by the Malawi's National AIDS Commission (NAC), a government agency responsible for oversight of HIV/AIDS funds and programming. In turn, NAC monitoring and evaluation of the country's AIDS programs was funded by the World Bank. The monitoring system was set up as a prerequisite to the implementation of the Global Fund grants for anti-retroviral treatment. According to Swidler, "African governments are dependent on and interpenetrated with international actors," which leads to programmatic and structural convergence in organizations. Yet local actors advance their own agendas through these relationships (Swidler, 2006, 271).

Swidler's analysis rings true with what I was told by media representatives. Father Saidi, a programmer of Radio Maria, a network of radio stations associated with the Catholic Church, said that they have organizations funding programs for different radio stations. Saidi said

> We have entered into a number of partnerships with some organizations whereby they are not buying airtime as such but they are giving us, say money, for production of programs. In a situation whereby we cannot manage to go where they want us to go have the program to meet people they want us to meet, then they have to provide [a] situation for that kind of thing... (Interview with Father Saidi, Mangochi, July 8, 2005)

It is difficult to know when one voice ends and another picks up. The interpenetration of NGOs, media, and government can be impossible to disentangle. Just as structural mandates by donors create what Swidler calls structural isomophism in AIDS organizations, these alliances, intersections, and relationships may lead to a partial convergence of messages and approaches.

Messages produced by NGOs, government, and media representatives tend to converge as well. In Malawi the public media, government, and donors tend to blame promiscuity and cultural practices for high rates of AIDS infection. According to Peters, Kambewa, and Walker, as AIDS became a major topic of newspapers, radio, and television from the mid-1990s to 2006 (along with sensational stories about witchcraft, corruption, sex, love, and crime) "[m]any articles condemned 'cultural practices,' a gloss for certain rituals involving sexual intercourse (such as at the end of initiation rites or after the death of a spouse and customs involving nonvoluntary sexual intercourse (such as 'widow inheritance')" (2010: 293). These "bad cultural practices" are in turn linked a failure of some to protect the rights of women.

My interviews with several media representatives in 2005 revealed that notions of civic education played into the messages surrounded health- and gender-related conflicts. Representatives of *The Nation*, Radio Maria, and MBC told me that after the advent of multiparty democracy one role of the media is to inform the public of their rights and the importance of not violating the rights of others. Excerpts from my interview with Father Saidi of Radio Maria again provide insight into the phenomenon:

> Say in family program [the station's program on issues relating to family life] you have the problem of say a woman who is ill treated by her husband in the name of cultural values, according to culture values so we say, no this is not, this is not the way . . . whereby somebody who's suffering she cannot come out to say that she is suffering because she has been taught to respect the husband. We bring out some of these issues to the general public's attention, to the attention of the general public through radio programming . . . as much as we have preserved the cultural values but we have also to see the issues of equality, gender equality and the like . . . there is a certain group that is making a kind of critical reflection in the society whereas the rest of the group is just down there-they're abiding by the cultural practices. They are abiding by them. They are saying, no, our forefathers used to do this way and we'll do the things in the same way. We cannot change. But now there are people who are reflecting on these cultural values to say, no, when [they] are beaten—it's a question of being beaten and you cannot call the husband—the police. It's a clear status to be brought to the police, it's not a question of tradition that you abide by whatever the husband says. If it is undemocratic you have to say it's not something that goes with an idea of equal dignity and equal rights so we have to say in a way our programs are informative to let the people—to share information with the people and then when they acquire this kind of information they can make their own assessment of the whole situation. They can critically analyze their cultural values. They can still be maintained. What can still be maintained and what can be dropped out as undemocratic . . . For instance in the lower part of our country Nsanje, there are some cultural practices they call it *kulowa kufa chokolo* whereby the husband or a gentleman inherits a wife of a brother or an uncle. These were the traditions that had been followed in the past but now people are coming in with the issue of the HIV/AIDS and saying, we cannot maintain this kind of practice. It's killing. So it's up to the people if they're informed—well—then they can make their own critical analysis of cultural practice. (Interview with Father Saidi, Mangochi, July 9, 2005)

The alliance of elite voices represented by the government, media, and NGOs sometimes create a disconnect with the everyday concerns of their listeners and creates an "us" (a certain group) and "them" (the rest of the group down there) dichotomy. They often focus disproportionately on "exotic" customs to the neglect of more "ordinary sexual relations" (Peters et al., 2010: 294). Yet, the words of Father Saidi demonstrate that when everyday sexual relations are discussed they may be framed as being highly problematic "culture" alongside the more "exotic" traditions. Such messages may be potentially alienating to portions of Malawi's population.

But messages about AIDS are "everywhere" in Malawi, and it is not only the government, NGOs, and media that are responsible for creating and disseminating them. Alternate sources of knowledge for navigating the epidemic are found within communities. Unofficial sources take up where official sources have been found lacking, suspect, or of limited practical utility.

Rumors and Epidemics

According to Gary Alan Fine, "Major epidemics have always provided a rich vein of folklore—particularly the creation of rumors, legends, folk beliefs and even humor. Accounts of cholera, polio and the Black Plague have demonstrated the connection of folklore to the popular understanding of disease" (1992: 69). In other words, by paying attention to informal communication relating to a disease, we can learn about a community's vernacular health beliefs. The folklore genres we are most concerned with here are those speculative genres common to everyday conversations whose purpose is to represent observed reality and fill in gaps for that which cannot be observed. Gossip and rumor obviously fit into this category of narrative.

Stewart and Strathern offer useful definitions of gossip and rumor. Gossip, which is talk about an absent subject, "takes place mutually among people in networks or groups. Rumor is unsubstantiated information, true or untrue, that passes by word of mouth, often in wider networks than gossip" (Stewart and Strathern, 2004: 38). While rumor or gossip can contain positive or negative judgments or characterization of their subject, people often linger over the negatives, the scandalous. In addition, it is important to note that practical advice, given explicitly or communicated implicitly, also flows from these exchanges.[13]

The notion of passing along and seeking information of "practical" value is of particular importance in the context of an epidemic disease like AIDS. This inevitably fatal, sexually transmitted disease, often undetected in the first years of its incubation, seems designed to spark speculation. In Malawi, when people get together to chat, they share observations and collectively construct the sexual histories of neighbors and relatives. They infer HIV serostatus of others through these sexual histories and sometimes use this information in choosing sexual partners (Kaler, 2004a; Poulin, 2007; Reniers, 2003; 2005; Schatz, 2002; Watkins, 2004). Sociologist Tamotsu Shibutani (1966) says that rumors arise in ambiguous situations, often some kind of crisis in which people pool their information in order to solve a problem. Rumor can thus form a basis for action. Speculation about the sexual histories of neighbors and relatives often functions as a preventative measure, forming a response to the problem of a possibly hidden disease. This preventative stance toward HIV is at odds with the portrayal of Africans in AIDS endemic areas as fatalistic with regards to AIDS (Campbell, 2003). Instead, people seek and pass along information that may help them navigate the epidemic.

By stating that gossip, rumor, and conspiracy theory may serve the function of educating people about the potential dangers of certain sexual partners or classes of "at risk" people, I do not suggest this is the only function they serve. In Ruth Finnegan's monograph *Oral Literature in Africa,* she criticizes the tendency of researchers of African prose narratives to assume that their primary function is to educate and socialize (1970: 330). This structural-functionalist paradigm was not only common in folktale analysis but also in the study of gossip. Max Gluckman, coming from the School of Structural Functionalism, analyzed gossip as a means by which group solidarity was created, social norms restated, and undesirable behaviors sanctioned. In other words, the integrity of social institutions is maintained through these discursive processes (Gluckman, 1963). Detractors were not far behind in firing their ripostes. Robert Paine says gossip is a competition of information transmission whereby a person creates a favorable impression of himself while degrading the reputation of a rival (Paine, 1967).

However, according to Abrahams, gossip is used for both enhancement of personal power as well as the articulation of community ideals. In his treatise "The Performance-Centered Approach to Gossip" he concludes that gossip, in that it encompasses these multiple functions, is related to other rhetorical strategies and genres (1970). For example, among the Vincentian speakers of English creole in the British West Indies, the equivalent of gossip "*commess*" was also related to joking, arguing, and ritualized performances. Similarly, everyday discussions of anxiety about AIDS treatment and prevention are registered across the related genres of rumor, gossip, urban/contemporary legend, and advice exchange. I would also add that these kinds of discourses, stirred up in the midst of worry and uncertainty, are linked to traditional practices in managing relations to family and state. Both the verbal and practical are parts of the self-same folk repertoire.

In a statement echoing that of Abrahams' above, Sally Engle Merry suggests that the conflict between the two modes—system centered and actor centered—could be resolved through a synthesis that opens up the way for further inquiry into the functions of rumors. She asserts that alone each perspective creates a caricature of reality. Not all gossip contributes to social equilibrium, nor is every instance of gossip about self-promotion (Merry, 1984). My analysis, which follows, is enriched by the notion of gossip as egocentric interest (i.e., self-promotion and disease avoidance) as well as the notion of gossip's function in articulating and reforming social norms.

In contrast, I hope to better understand the imagined worlds, shared values, and practical wisdom of my informants through the study of gossip and related genres. However, the construction of moral characters remains a central activity of gossip examined here because a person's reputation plays a role in strategies of exclusion.

If rumor is an instance of collective belief formation then in Malawi the discursive culmination of that collective belief formation is advice.[14] Indeed, advice is often said to be "good medicine," and girls in Northern Malawi pay a small fee for the advice they receive from elders at their menstrual initiation. Throughout the early years of their marriages they continue to receive counsel. So while rumor seeks to inform and reveal hidden truths, it is advice that explicitly translates that information into a script for action. Advice often flows vertically from elder generations to younger generations, but it can also flow laterally between agemates and friends.

I draw upon Luise White's approach to the vampire narratives circulating in colonial East and Central Africa to structure my analysis. White conceives of these narratives about the experiences of colonial medicine as neither true nor false, neither depictions of actual events nor fantasies of irrational minds, but rather as descriptions of "meanings and powers and ideas" informing the ways people behave and think (White, 2000: 89). She suggests such stories should be read for generic, formulaic qualities. In particular, White finds that vampire rumors, when juxtaposed to triumphant tales of biomedical practice, can illuminate the context in which biomedicine was practiced in colonial East and Central Africa (2000: 89). The same can be said of current contemporary legends (sometimes called "urban legends"), which abound in Malawi.

Several scholars have linked conspiracy rumors, contemporary legends, and witchcraft accusations to the processes of democratization and the monetization and globalizing of economic systems (Ashforth, 1996; Auslander, 1993; Comaroff and Comaroff, 1993; Geschiere, 1997; Sanders, 2003; West and Luedke, 2006). The resultant "malcontents of modernity" (Comaroff and Comaroff, 1993) include the experience of entrenched poverty and the exacerbation of political, economic, gender, and health disparities on local and global scales. Some scholars have noted that the AIDS epidemic has spurred witchcraft accusations in Haiti and Southern Africa as people try to make sense of misfortune, avoid being labeled as diseased, and interpret illness symptoms with respect to familiar etiological theories (Ashforth, 2002; 2005; Farmer, 1992; Rödlach, 2006; Stadler, 2003; Yamba, 1997). My reference to witchcraft is a variation on the notion that the new (in this case AIDS) is interpreted in the light of the old, familiar idioms of suspicion and accusation. In Malawian cosmology, the sacred or spiritual (good and bad) is not far from the experience of everyday life and indeed breaks into everyday life on a regular basis. Thus the stories of the mundane (advice, gossip, and fighting) outlined in the first chapters of the book are not part of a reality distinct from the world envisioned by the rumors and legends of the supernatural in the latter part of the book.

Chapter 2 investigates ways that married women in rural Northern Malawi struggle to reduce HIV risk introduced by potentially unfaithful husbands through an assortment of strategies handed down from elders and friends and communicated in daily talk: rumor, counseling, joking, gossiping, commiserating, and complaining. Malawians go beyond individualistic public health recommendations for AIDS prevention of the ABCs. Some of the creative strategies women employ in HIV prevention are aimed at changing the behaviors of others. Drawing on a combination of interviews and ethnographic reports from local informants, this chapter explores women's efforts to secure fidelity with actions directed toward altering their husbands' extramarital sexual practices.

When describing their expectations and experiences of marriage, Malawian women say, "marriage is endurance." Yet the idea of endurance is multifaceted, signifying diverse ways of thriving, coping, surviving, and adapting. Central to women's responses to marital insecurity are informal communication and folk knowledge (lore). This chapter introduces common responses of Northern Malawian women to common marital conflicts. Some techniques of conflict negotiation take part in reshaping gender roles, while others are essentially conservative.

In their efforts to ensure fidelity of their spouses, some women in rural Malawi resort to challenging female rivals, that is, the "other" woman in their husbands' lives. Chapter 3 examines these challenges, which I describe as "aggressive" which can take the form of physical aggression or social aggression. The aim of either type is to force the "other woman" away from the contested husband and from the village if possible. Women use aggressive strategies for several reasons. Sometimes they resort to aggression when other tactics for more directly influencing the fidelity of their spouses fail. As described in chapter 2, women go to elders and go-betweens for advice and intervention and are often told to counsel their husbands or bring their husbands to the elders for counseling. These tactics and others like them do not always yield the desired results. Aggressive tactics are also used when women wish to avoid uncomfortable or dangerous confrontations with husbands. In other words, an inability to direct the behavior of a spouse can precipitate the use of unorthodox, aggressive strategies of physical violence or social aggression. Tales of infidelity and aggressive confrontation are seen as highly entertaining and yet simultaneously sad or shameful.

In chapter 3, I present narratives of wives challenging sexual rivals to discern what social structures and maneuvers contribute to the relative success or failure of aggressive strategies. My analysis of fight narratives reveals the importance of processes of labeling and exclusion in aggressive strategies. Even physical attacks build upon discourses to stigmatize and label sexual rivals as threats to the health of the community. Yet interviews and ethnographic journals reveal that seldom is the "outsider," marginal identity of a rival firmly fixed within a community. Communities harbor the uneasy sense that woman against woman confrontations are at once a kind of collective or vicarious catharsis and a shameful, morally questionable opposition of vulnerable woman against vulnerable woman. These tales are "funny yet sorrowful."

In 2008, a rumor began to circulate claiming that in the Southern Malawi city of Zomba, a new sexually transmitted disease was emerging. This disease, *mphutsi* (maggot), was said to be more dangerous than AIDS because it kills faster. In particular it was said to kill men faster than women and was believed to be more difficult to treat in men than women. Journalists reported that men were becoming angry with prostitutes in some cities and shouting at them, blaming them for spreading the disease. In chapter 4, I analyze stories about *mphutsi* with an eye to discerning what makes them plausible and the reasons the disease provoked such terror.

The plausibility of a rumor is related to prior knowledge and experience of the community in which the information is circulating. Plausibility is a function of cultural context—the imagery, epistemology, and expectation of a given community. While the experience and knowledge of various STIs (sexually transmitted infections) form the general epistemological groundwork for incorporating tales of a new disease. I argue that the entrenchment and comprehensive impact of AIDS makes it the primary point of reference for new STIs; HIV/AIDS, therefore, is a primary lens through which to interpret plausibility of *mphutsi*. Stories of *mphutsi* shed light on evolving attitudes about AIDS in a time when drug treatment is more widely available than ever. In contrast to HIV, which is hidden by a prolonged incubation period and then with medicine, *mphutsi* provokes both a sense of terror and relief. The ability to easily diagnose the disease and identify categories of "diseased" or "at risk" groups is a rarity in a society where one of the most deadly diseases is generalized and obscured from view. The chapter also confirms the notion put forth by some that HIV/AIDS has been established as a fact of life, a new norm to which societies have adjusted. On one level *mphutsi* tales function as indictments of mobile women who are seen as voracious sexual aggressors spreading a disease that literally eats a man to death. At the same time, they indicate women's vulnerability. The themes in this tale echo concerns expressed in the chapter Funny Yet Sorrowful; are women victims or aggressors?

In chapter 5, I analyze motifs of Malawian stories of sorcerer-seducers within the milieu of a high HIV/AIDS prevalence, gendered struggles over sexuality within marriage, and regionally popular supernatural assault and possession tales. Night holds peculiar terrors for women in Malawian households as they lie in their beds. It is said that in the night some men use charms to seduce women as they sleep. In 2005, fear of these stealth seducers rose to a high level when girls from a secondary school reported such attacks. Anxious students asked, "Can girls contract AIDS from one of these attacks?" Older women also fear attacks of this sort. Some married women sleeping next to their husbands claim to have been overcome by witches.

A popular motif in Southern and Central Africa is that of people who, as they sleep, are magically made to work in others' gardens. They wake to find themselves drained of energy. In other words, people become part of a zombie workforce that has lost its agency. Their bodies come under the control of others. A similar loss of control of the body is evident in the supernatural attack tales in which women are paralyzed or sleeping while under sexual attack. Fear of contracting AIDS adds another layer of concern. The motif of being drained of energy reaches its extreme in the fear of AIDS. What can more efficiently drain someone of life than AIDS, a disease that is said in Malawi to make people "dead but alive" and render them "the walking dead?"

These narratives that speak to a gendered experience of helplessness and vulnerability echo throughout the region and dramatize the media-fed notion of a gender battle sparked by efforts of international human rights organizations. Young women who have collective fantasies of phantom rape are not so much dreaming of an initiation into their lives as sexual beings; but rather they are being initiated into lives of violated sexuality. In these stories even husbands have not been able to stop men from stealing sex from their wives. Indeed, sometimes they are there when it is happening.

In a country where "advice is good medicine" and "there is no secret under the sun," the power of informal discourse is appreciated as a valuable mode of knowing, social critique, and basis for action. Each chapter showcases different ways of uncovering hidden knowledge. In chapter 2, I show how women gather information and advice to influence the actions of "wayward" husbands, judiciously revealing the gleaned information to those who may support their cause. Indeed, the advice and the power of revealing secrets have much in common with Malawian notions of healing medicine. A major function of traditional healing diviners is to uncover who is responsible for someone's sickness. One respondent sought a love potion that would cause her husband to reveal his lover's name. In chapter 3, I show how women take hold of story and propel certain images of themselves and their rivals through the community to carve out a position for themselves. Even in examining stories circulating on a larger scale the power of hidden knowledge revealed is apparent. *Mphutsi* stories of a spectacularly visible sexually transmitted disease suggest a wariness of increasingly hidden HIV status in the emerging era of biomedical AIDS treatment in Malawi. At the same time, they reveal the desire for easy categorization of who is at risk and who is not. Finally, *mgoneko* stories speak to the abuse that takes place behind closed doors in marriages, initiation, and in schools. Alongside the media light shed on the problem of domestic abuse and gender-based violence of various kinds, the *mgoneko* rumors add a popular voice to the cacophony, revealing women's sense of vulnerability and couching the critique in terms that calls for greater intervention.

CHAPTER 2

ADVICE IS GOOD MEDICINE: MARRIAGE, ADVICE, AND THE COMFORTS OF HOME

During my first week in the Rumphi District of Malawi, I met Patricia. She and two other women were laughingly commiserating about marital problems as Catherine and I tagged along. Patricia, a woman in her 30s, was complaining about her husband, who had been missing for eleven days. She had heard and believed that he was with his girlfriend in a nearby shantytown. Her friends murmured their sympathy, and we piled into a car and drove to a convenience store, where she continued to complain as we waited in the parking lot for one of the women to emerge from the store. Patricia turned to me, eyes gleaming through the shadows, and said with a laugh, "Marriage is one way to get AIDS. The man—even if he's fine at first—he changes. Though you don't move around. He'll just bring it to you as a gift and you will just receive it—happily—open arms and open legs!" (Wilson fieldnotes, November 27, 2005) We all laughed in that moment, but I could still remember her frustrated tears from the afternoon when the women had gathered around her in her home. That conversation, occurring within the first weeks of my arrival in Malawi, compelled me to ask: What prevention strategies do wives in Malawi employ when they feel at risk of contracting AIDS from their husbands, and what role does the commiseration and counsel of others, especially women, play in devising those tactics?

The purpose of this chapter and the next is to investigate ways in which married women in rural Northern Malawi struggle to reduce HIV risk introduced by potentially unfaithful husbands through an assortment of strategies handed down from elders and friends and communicated in daily talk: rumor, counseling, joking, gossiping, commiserating, and complaining. Malawians utilize numerous strategies for AIDS prevention beyond the ABCs (Abstain, Be Faithful, and Use Condoms) recommended in public health campaigns. Several creative strategies women employ in HIV prevention are aimed at changing the behaviors of another person. This chapter examines women's efforts to secure fidelity with actions directed toward changing their husbands' extramarital sexual practices rather than their own.

Worried Wives

Marriage has come under scrutiny as a potentially disempowering institution for women in contexts such as Malawi. From social science to international human rights organizations, women are presented as vulnerable and unable to enforce the use of condoms or live independently of a husband's cash income (Amaro, 1995; Baylies and Bujra, 2000; Doyal, 1995; Heise et al., 1995; Issiaka et al., 2001; Kandiyoti, 1988; Lesch and Kruger, 2005; Maman et al, 2001; McGrath et al., 1992; Seeley, 1994; Sinding, 2005). Indeed, quantitative studies suggest that, on average, women in Malawi are more worried about contracting AIDS than men are (Clark, 2005; Smith, 2003; Smith and Watkins, 2005). Not only are women more worried, their worry is of a different kind. Whereas men fear infection from extramarital partners, women are more afraid that their husbands will pass the disease on to them from girlfriends or other wives (Clark, 2005; Smith and Watkins, 2005).[1] They have reason to worry. Malawian men are far more likely to have extramarital partners than women. And although men are more likely to use condoms with extramarital partners than with their wives, the use of condoms is not consistent (NSO, 2005). This means that men who have unprotected sex with their extramarital partners increase the risk of the transmission of AIDS to their wives. So what can women do?

Both Enid Schatz (2002) and Georges Reniers (2003; 2006) have found that women in Malawi are beginning to use divorce as a strategy for removing themselves from risk of HIV infection when their husbands are unfaithful.[2] Divorce is not uncommon in Malawi. In Rumphi, 14 percent of first marriages have ended after five years. After 25 years about 40 percent of first marriages have ended (Reniers, 2006: 82). But divorce usually only takes place after a series of interventions have failed and is complicated by issues of child custody, financial constraints, *lobola* (bridewealth), [3] and various family obligations. In a patrilineal society like that of the Tumbuka, divorce is easier for a man to initiate than a woman. Children become part of the husband's kin group upon the payment of *lobola,* or an agreed-upon monetary bridewealth, and a woman may risk leaving them behind if she decides to leave the marriage; though, in the modified patrilineal practices of the Tumbuka, mothers of young children often maintain custody (Kerr, 2005a, 57). In addition, women lose access to the affinal lands they have cultivated. Besides these factors, the bonds of affection may keep a woman in a highly troubled marriage. Instead of divorcing, many Tumbuka women find themselves negotiating AIDS risk within the context of marriage and learning a variety of ways to endure.

Women's Strategies in Marital Conflict

Women in Southern Africa have long worked within the confines of patriarchal societies to exert influence on their situations. Elizabeth Schmidt, in her study of Shona women from 1870–1939, highlights the ways in which women exerted influence informally when their access to institutionalized power was lacking. Drawing on the distinction made by Bourque and Warren, Schmidt characterizes "power" as "the capacity to define and enforce the rules by which society is governed (1992: 20). Power is institutionalized and formalized, whereas "influence" consists of informal strategies used by those excluded from prominent institutions. The goal of these strategies is to "limit the power of others and the ways in which that power impinges upon their lives (1992: 20)." Furthermore, because they are systematically excluded from key institutions based on gender, women rely more exclusively on strategies of influence than men.

Schmidt notes that many of these strategies are culturally acceptable. Indeed, many of the strategies Schmidt enumerated are folkloric in nature, including gossip (which she describes as a means of social control) and subversive work songs. Other means of expressing displeasure in order to exert influence included the naming of children. Through the names of their children, cowives in a polygamous marriage would express displeasure with one another. The songs sung while women pounded maize were a means by which they could complain about the ill-treatment of their in-laws. Such traditions of complaint through song have also been documented in

Malawi (White, 1987; Friedson, 1996). Likewise, gossip and rumor are a means by which the Tumbuka women I interviewed assert influence and reshape their social contexts.

Because expert advice passed along official governmental public health channels does not adequately address popular desires to affect the behavior of dangerous others in their everyday lived realities, women (both spouses and sexual rivals) seek the expert advice of elders and knowledgeable peers from within their communities. Elders, in particular, are entrusted with "cultural authority" as defined by Hufford as a kind of authority derived from experience that compels others to trust (1996: 92). The system of familial council for marital problems relating to infidelity and AIDS is an "alternative institution" to more official institutions such as traditional healers and voluntary counseling and testing (VCT) at biomedical health centers. The exchanges among women and elders constitute a kind of folk family therapy which addresses more holistically the social situation in which women experience AIDS risk. Analysis of ethnographic data exposes the importance of rumor, gossip, and advice as a means by which women deal with vulnerability and find strength within social bounds of marriage and kin obligations. Furthermore, because cultural authorities often hold social authority, that is the "ability to compel obedience" based on "the belief that authority holds adequate power in reserve," women rely on them for both wise council and their ability to enforce decisions in a particular social sphere. Wives receive counsel when they are troubled by rumors of infidelity, including advice to confront their husbands, endure, pray, or use love potions. Not all stories or remedies are accepted at face value, but rather women question sources and motivations, testing gossip against their own observations and testing social remedies against their own experimentation.

The first section of this chapter outlines key elements of the cultural and social context of Tumbuka women's anti-adultery strategies. Among the elements discussed here are women's perception of AIDS risk from husbands, their reliance upon friends and neighbors to report spousal activities, and the problem of working out marital conflicts while living among in-laws and strangers. The next section presents women's accounts of what happens when they take their complaints to in-law elders. What advice is given and what impact do wives have when they act upon it? The last section also deals with advice but this time advice from peer group friends and natal relatives. When dissatisfied with counsel from in-laws, a woman may seek help from friends or family back home. The contrast between counsel from affinal elders and natal elders suggests the existence of competing orthodoxies for dealing with marital infidelity.

No Secret under the Sun

Infidelity is a common topic of gossip in Malawi provoking expressions of both the voyeuristic pleasure and moral outrage. In their conversations about adultery, people relish the idea that they have stumbled onto hidden knowledge of wrongdoings. They also enjoy making judgments about the adulterers, speculating as to motives and predicting consequences for the persons discussed and for the community as a whole.

This chapter draws upon informal conversations recorded in my field notes, in-depth interviews, and the field notes of trained journalers. Employing journalers expands the ethnographer's access to local knowledge and informal communications. Folklore scholars of urban legends have frequently relied upon students as collectors and ethnographers of urban legends in circulation within their own networks (i.e., Brunvand, 1981; Fine, 1992; Turner, 1993).

Journaler Hastings Mkandawire recounts a conversation that took place while waiting in line to buy maize. The buzz in line that morning was that the watchman at the ADMARC (Agricultural Development and Marketing Corporation) had allowed a woman to buy twice the rationed amount of maize in exchange for sleeping with him. Mkandawire summarizes the stories he heard from several people that morning and finishes his account with comments made by the friends with whom he was chatting. He begins by suggesting a motive for the woman's behavior saying,

> People used so many tactics on this day to secure enough maize for their families. One strange tactic was the one I got on the day when we were on the queue struggling to buy 10 kgs of Maize. A certain woman from Mpaka happened to have a good terms with one of the workers at the Admarc, the watchman. The watchmen then assured her that if she wanted to get enough kgs the following day she should accept to do sex with him. Considering the extent of the famine in her family the woman accepted to do that with the watchman the same Sunday night. Before Monday everything was done. The watchman

> assured the woman to be among the first people to be served that morning she was also told that she will have an additional 10kgs on top of the recommended 10kgs as saying goes there is no secret under the sun some body who went out to urin[ate] behind the Admarc saw... their agreement as usual [a] secret is only between two people this third person was the one who started telling people at the Admarc Major was now explaining to people as if the one who got the first hand information.
>
> *Major*: You are now telling us only 10kgs but our friends who gave her body to you got 25kgs right from the same Admarc this is not fare [sic].
>
> *Hastings*: You mean others were getting 25kgs right from here?
>
> *Major*: Only one lady has gone out with this place with 25kgs of maize on the special offer.
>
> *Mary Luwemba*: What our friend has done is useless, if its because of famine that has befallen into Malawi it better for us to die than to do sex with somebody you don't know for the sake of having 25kgs of maize the AIDS worries me much. (Mkandawire research journal, February 2006)

The proverbial phrase "There is no secret under the sun" is common throughout Malawi and is sometimes used to punctuate stories of scandalous secrets revealed. Two broad but related interpretations suggest themselves.[4] One speaks to the inevitability of truth being revealed. Everything that has been done in secret will be known. This interpretation begs the question: How will the secrets be revealed? The second interpretation addresses this question. "No secret under the sun" implies the presence of knowing subjects, people who know information that is being hidden. Sometimes women are suspicious of infidelity through their own observations. For them the secret is "revealed" by frequent and poorly justified absences of their husbands. In these cases they are the knowing subjects, but often knowledge of a spouse's extramarital activities is revealed or confirmed by other people—neighbors, friends, and relatives.

General fears of secret affairs as expressed by Mrs. Luwemba can be contrasted with personal and specific fears for the cuckolded spouse. When a woman is told that her husband has been spotted with another woman, she heeds these particular stories with a greater level of attention. During our interview Kondwani Kwenda recounted the multiple ways in which she learned of her husband's infidelity (February 2, 2006). The following exchange took place between Kondwani and my research assistant, Catherine Simkonda, during an interview:

K: When I was six months pregnant my husband had a girlfriend here, he still continued with her [during the pregnancy].
C: With all that beauty? [Catherine referred to the respondent's appearance]
K: When I was seven she was four months pregnant also. When I was eight I delivered at eight. He gave her money for abortion at five months... He gave her K500 for abortion. When he was doing this I didn't know.
C: Not even partial?
K: Not even that, I didn't know. I was at the hospital delivering. I was delivering the child which died...
C: So after you delivered how long did it take before you knew?
K: After the child died I delivered on 13th April and he died on 19th May. So I heard the story in July... After I was cleansed and we started sleeping together it was when I heard.
C: Who said this? Who told you?
K: It was my mother. She heard this at the funeral of my child. [unintelligible]
C: Your own mother?
K: Yes...
C: So did you ask him?
K: I did and he denied it. Another person told me again. He said they were just loving each other. I asked him he denied it again.

Later on, after Kondwani stopped drawing and warming water for his bath, cooking for him regularly, or sleeping with him, her husband confessed and apologized, saying he did not know what he was doing. Kondwani, like other women, took the rumors seriously enough to investigate further.

Interventions begin with the investigation of a rumor. Such was the case for Kettie Harawa when she heard that her husband was proposing other women.[5] Her neighbor, who related to us the same story, cautioned her not to accept the story at face value but to prove it. So, according to Kettie, she followed her husband one day to "prove" the story and saw him chatting with the young woman. Kettie hid behind the bush to listen in on their conversation. Later she complained about the issue to his aunt and brought him to the elders to be counseled.

"They Say That Staying in Marriage Is Endurance"

Why is it so important to "prove" the rumors?[6] Part of the need to prove a story stems from a woman's position in her virilocal setting. Several women told me that before they relocated to their husband's village, they were warned by their elders back home that on your new compound you may find people who speak badly about you and tell lies. The women I interviewed were told to remain quiet. Ruth Chirwa said, "*Wakutenga kukhala pa nthengwa nkupilira*" ["To stay in marriage is endurance."]. When you marry, you may find rude people at your compound treating you poorly "because they can say a lot of bad things since it is not your home, just keep it in your heart. Do not talk anyhow" (January 12, 2006).[7] In virilocal Tumbukaland women say, "I am a stranger here" or "I am new here" when they come to their husbands' compounds, and because of this they may be reluctant to speak up in what may be a hostile territory.[8] Elders in their natal villages prepare women for the possibility of discomfort or even hostility in their marital homes. Women expressed the most fear of being overworked at the service of in-laws, being talked about badly, and being beaten by husbands. The ubiquity of the experience of a harsh welcome into a marital village is evidenced by a folktale widespread throughout sub-Saharan Africa.

Boyd and Fardon (1998) analyze several versions of a folktale they call "The girl who wanted an unblemished husband," in which a girl spurns all suitors except the one found to be without physical blemish. Typically the plot unfolds as follows: against the judgment of her elders, a girl marries a physically flawless man and follows him to his village only to find there that she has been deceived. Her husband has been disguised, and after marriage he transforms into his true form, a leprous and grotesque man or else a hideous monster. In some versions the man is a cannibal, and he and his friends plot to consume the woman. The bride escapes but finds herself in the wilderness, stuck high in a tree and surrounded by threatening in-laws. She wards off the danger with singing and is later rescued, ultimately returning to her natal village to safety. In other versions of the story, a woman is accompanied to her marital village by a younger sister who discovers the hidden monstrous nature of her sister's husband and warns her sister not to "eat," that is, have sexual intercourse with her husband (Bill, 1994).[9] Most versions of the tale end with the girl fleeing the marital village for her natal home. I refer to this folktale occasionally in my analysis of women's kin-based prevention strategies, looking upon it as a kind of vocabulary or template for women's experiences in marriage.

One explicit moral of the story enjoins brides to hear the advice of elders, silently endure when prudent, and look through the obvious to discover the hidden nature of things. In other words, when one is among strangers, do not trust everything you hear or see—you may be deceived. Constance Mzumala told us that some women will lie about another woman's husband if they like him themselves. There was a married man who used to buy fish in Phukwa from a certain woman, she said, and they would greet each other cheerfully during these encounters. A woman who observed their interactions went to the man's wife and said the two were having an affair. The wife did not believe her because she had another friend in Phukwa (a pseudonym for a nearby marketplace) who told her otherwise. The wife criticized the talebearer, telling her, "Never to do it again because you can let people kill each other." In other words, the stories can promote quarrels that can escalate to violence.

Despite the danger, women rely on each other for information. When we asked this same Constance Mzumala how one could know her husband was cheating, she told us, "Not all people will hate you." Your friends will tell you about your husband's infidelity "and you will find they like going to Phukwa!"[10] Surveillance conducted through a network of friends or sisters-in-law was common among the women we interviewed. Elizabeth Mkandawire, who was 20 years old with a newborn, said she was worried about her husband's movements. She said, "My husband stays in Mhuju and he is a driver, so I hear a lot of stories saying he is proposing so and so and so." She believes the people telling her the stories but is unable to investigate on her own. Elizabeth said, "As I stay here, it is difficult. Sometimes I want to do that [investigate]," but instead all her information is derived from hearsay rather than direct observation. Elizabeth's story demonstrates extreme reliance upon a network to reveal what is hidden under the sun or by distance.

The aphorism "marriage is endurance" was expressed not only in the context of living among demanding or troublemaking in-laws but also when women referred to ways in which men could (as in the folktale) change after marriage.[11] Women expressed the most fear that men would stop "hoeing," that is, working hard to provide materials for the family, or that they would beat them "harshly" or "unnecessarily." Secondarily, women worried that a man would start having girlfriends or acquire a new wife. They were advised by elders at home, elders in the new villages, and by agemate friends that if a husband changes, you ought to endure these negative transformations. Some believed that these transformations are inevitable. One of the middle-aged women we spoke to said that nowadays complaints about cheating and polygamy are routine. She warns younger women, "When you marry, don't think you are alone" (Estery Gondwe, January 10, 2006). Olifa Mhango said, "My mum told me that every man changes, so just endure."

What do these women mean when they say you must endure? Selina Mweso (age 20) explained, "Whether he will have a girl, you should endure, whether he beats you, whether he is bad just endure" (February 2, 2006). Her exegesis encompassed what one endures but not how to endure it. In practical terms, enduring could signify different actions and goals. The most basic meaning of enduring marriage is to "just stay," that is, to not go home. Beyond continued presence in the marital home, enduring for some is passive and for others is highly active. Several elders told women to be patient if they found out their husbands were cheating. Don't react in anger and get into a fight but wait to "hear more" so that your reactions may be tailored to the situation and so that you might not find yourself abandoned for "overreacting." *Agogo* Fanny Ngwira[12] said when faced with the problem of an unfaithful husband, "The real medicine is cooking and hoeing"; in other words, continuing to take care of the house and the husband's sexual needs. In the end he may return to you, the steadfast, hardworking, and calm wife, and abandon the other woman for, "[I]f you are two [wives], you will get the disease [AIDS]," said Agness Kumwenda.

Among elders there is a strong orientation to urge their young in-laws to endure, that is, to persevere in marriage. The day before we met with Lusungu Kayira; a young in-law had visited her to complain and get bus fare to travel home. The young woman wanted to go back home because her husband was trying to bring another woman into the marriage. He even insisted that she go with him to collect the new wife.[13] He told his wife that if she did not listen then she was disobeying his rules, as if to imply that he would punish her in some way. Lusungu described the young woman as depressed because her polygynous husband was no longer providing food to the household. However, Lusungu did not give the woman money to go home. Instead, she told the girl to speak to her father-in-law. We asked Lusungu what she expected the father-in-law to say. "What can he say?" she replied. "He is the father of the husband, he will tell her to stay." Despite the sympathy she felt toward the young woman and all she had experienced, Lusungu recommended endurance in solidarity with the will of her husband's relatives.

Endurance, as I have described thus far, has been decidedly passive, but some women practice what I call "active endurance." When Ruth Chirwa said marriage is endurance, she followed the adage with an inventory of the troubles she has encountered and the strategies with which she met those challenges. Upon hearing that her husband was contemplating marrying another woman, she sought advice, confronted him, followed him, used love potions, prayed, took him to church—and finally drove the other woman out of the village.[14] Kondwani Kwenda spoke of a similar kind of endurance when she talked about punishing her husband by refusing to "cook" for him, both literally and figuratively.[15] While Kondwani punished her husband, she said they were not living "free," that is, they were together in a state of dis-ease until he confessed and apologized. It is at that turning point of confession and apology that Kondwani inserted her comment that marriage is endurance. I present Kondwani's and Ruth's actions as examples of active endurance.

The alternative to enduring is to go home or ultimately to divorce, but for some there does not seem much point to divorcing a "mobile" husband because it is likely that this man has already transmitted HIV to them. Mrs. Chavula told us that when young women come complaining about their husbands' movements, fearing AIDS, she tells them to just endure, because if their husband is infected then they are infected as well. Agness Kumwenda said a woman came to her to complain about a husband who had married his brother's widow. She had no advice to offer to the woman. Mrs. Kumwenda said, "Nowadays many people are complaining and say 'Ah ah, we already know we have AIDS. We already know.'" We asked Mrs. Kumwenda what her friend was doing about the situation. "The woman is now staying with her husband, but she has said to him, 'Your brother died of AIDS, so are we not dying also? We have already died. As of now the widow is dead. Are we going to live longer? We are finished.'" She had no advice to offer the woman; as far as she could see the damage had already been done.

Complaints about mobile husbands are common, says Tamora Gondwe. Wives say to her,

> "My husband will take the disease—he is not moving well." When we answer them we say, "Oh yes, he will get the disease." The badness is that they are not known. When you say you are infected because this virus [it] eats you slowly—sometimes 5 years can pass. Because you will not know when you slept with somebody who was infected. She will just say "It's my husband you don't refuse him." You [as an advisor] will just discuss that you are sick, Your blood is infected. And you start feeling unwell, whether you or your husband. But if you know, well...

The last two quotes exemplify several aspects of the popular beliefs about AIDS in Malawi. Generally speaking, people overestimate how easy it is to get AIDS and tend to think that one sexual encounter with an HIV-positive partner means that the disease was certainly transmitted. When this belief is extended to regular partners such as spouses then people speak with even greater conviction that if the husband has HIV then the wife definitely has it, and vice versa. The certainty of these beliefs about the ease with which the disease is transmitted is hedged by the fact that many people do not get tested for HIV or know for certain the HIV status of their husbands or their husbands' partners. The gap of certainty contains the kernel of hope that preventive action is still possible for those who are not certain of their status.

Endurance is not idle resignation or stoicism but for many people is an active resolve to make use of the knowledge and resources within their communities and within themselves. Endurance, therefore, rests not on fatalism but upon hope that change may be possible. When women are faced with criticisms of laziness, they work harder; when faced with rumors of unfaithful husbands, they listen to "hear more." The next section examines what it means to "hear more."

Advice Is Good Medicine

In 2004, when I spent time in Southern Malawi at a roadside hair salon, the young woman who ran the business asked me if I had any medicine for her business. I was confused until my interpreter explained that she wants advice. "Advice is good medicine" she told me. Malawians seek literal *mankhwala*, that is, medicine, for financial, interpersonal, and physical health. The *mankhwala* of advice is an additional or complementary type of medicine Malawians seek.

In Tumbukaland, before a woman joins her husband at his compound, she receives advice from her aunts and, less formally, from her friends. Once she is living in her husband's compound, she is expected to go to elders of her husband's family for advice in domestic matters—both in keeping the house and in all manner of marital conflicts that may and do arise. We asked some female elders what advice they gave out to the young women who came to them seeking advice and counsel. Problems brought to them included struggles over finances, infidelity, drinking habits, and the execution of household chores.

Joyce Mhango told us she had to criticize her granddaughter-in-law because she was not bringing bathing water to her husband and the meals she cooked were slow in coming. In annoyance, he retaliated by withholding money when the granddaughter-in-law asked for cash to buy household goods. When Mrs. Mhango sat down with the young woman, she asked, "Did they advise you at home [about] who is the head of the family? You are under the man. But what you are talking is good. When he is talking bad, criticize him. If he is not listening, come to me"(January 27, 2006). "Criticize him" or "confront him calmly" was also the advice that most of the young women heard when they complained to the elder women about their husband's infidelity. Women were told to advise their husbands about the perils of their bad behavior, and if that did not work, ask the elders to speak to him—to counsel him. The repetition of these three steps in advice in marital problem solving—complain, confront, and bring your spouse for counsel—could be said to make up an idealized sequence. The point of counsel is that the so-called bad behavior should change, but not everyone has faith that change is possible.

One elder women spoke with despair about the men who were going out with bar girls. And then of women who sleep with men for financial support. She laments that AIDS will kill these men and women.

> *R*: I even tell them that—"Don't go there, you children. Look that one lost her husband so you will be going out with her, you will die... They don't listen.

I: Have you ever seen anyone advised who has changed?
R: Oh no, they don't change. They [women] love them because they will eat good food, so they cannot change. They cannot stop. Because it is nice. So they cannot change even if you say, "Sit down my child;" they say, "you old people you are troublesome." So when you are talking they say that – "Old timers – this is new," so they just continue. Time does not pass, they just die. (Tembo, January 12, 2006)

Young women are often counseled by elders not to enter into sexual relationships with men in order to gain financial support. In "When They See Money They Think It's Life: Money, Modernity and Morality in Two Sites in Rural Malawi," Amy Kaler writes that elders believe young women are "going to the grave" by chasing men who provide gifts and money (Kaler, 2006). Elders claim that the temptation to become involved with men with cash causes women, single or married, to ignore their advice.

In a similar elders' lament, Estery Gondwe told us that she doesn't dare try to advise some of the young people she sees nowadays. Now men will insult you if you try to interfere, she said.[16] Her advice to fearful wives is for them to endure the cheating of their husbands because some men will recognize the error of their ways and come back on their own. What is implied is that others will not.[17]

Giving and receiving advice is perceived as an important means for establishing "healthy" social norms. The conversation below takes place between Hastings, an elderly neighbor, Mrs. Mbale, and her relatives.

Mrs. Mbale [a woman in her 70s]: [It is] true that [the] young girl you see, she has seen a lot of things more [than] what I have seen in the world. Before her first marriage she was being beaten by wives of the husbands she was going out with, going into marriage we thought, people of Luwagha will be relieved [of] her bad habit. While in the marriage she was still going out of the marriage circle till she was discovered hence the end of the first marriage.

She was been exchanging men as if they are clothes, Now if the mission is that of going into marriage then she has gone to the No. 5 husband. She must have a certain mission to fulfill.

Alex [a teen and relative of Mrs. Mbale]: She has got a mission of tast[ing] all men in the country..." We all laughed at the joke which Alex fixed on.

In Malawi, the belief that innocent people can suffer sickness because of the wrongdoings of others is a part of the Malawian conceptions of disease pre-dating the advent of AIDS. According to Morris, literature on African disease concepts have identified four broad categories of disease causation, which are also evident among the Chewa of Southern Malawi: natural diseases or those "from God," those deriving from moral infringement, afflictions caused by witchcraft or sorcery (*matsenga*, that is, magic), and spirit induced afflictions (Morris 1996; Peters, Kambewa, and Walker, 2008). Illnesses caused by a violation of some ritual or moral interdiction are said to cause suffering to those connected to the violators. A few examples of such diseases include *tsempho*, *likango*, and *ndaka* (Morris, 1996: 130). In particular, ideas about the cause of *tsempho* (also called *mdulo*) seem to bear a strong resemblance to ideas expressed about both AIDS and *mphutsi*. Morris describes the disease as follows: "It is considered to be a particular kind of wasting disease which may have fatal consequences if counter-measures are not taken in the form of medicines. The disease is related to promiscuous sexual relationships, or to indulging in sexual intercourse by spouses during ritually prohibited periods. The disease affects men, women, and young children, and is caused by another's transgression." (Morris, 1996: 132). In chapter 3, where I write about women who seek to separate their husbands' from extramarital partners, I make a similar observation. Although some women try to label others as morally and physically sick and thus a danger to the community, it is difficult to make these stigmatizing labels stick because people can easily picture themselves in the same problems as the potentially stigmatized individual. Hastings: "Sister, do you know that the dog ate shit because it lacked advice?" That girl can change if she can be properly advised on what she is doing. People have changed their bad habits after being advised properly.

Mrs. Gondwe [the daughter of Mrs. Mbale]:

> "Advisors were there at her home but [she] didn't want to take use of all the advise [sic] people were advising her. Now she is affected with a deadly disease she had loosened." (Mkandawire research journal, February 2006)

This excerpt reveals the value placed on receiving wise counsel. Behavior, in emic terms, is directly related to the counsel one has received. Without "proper" advice one can participate in risky, undesirable behavior—one can eat shit rather than the good medicine of advice. Implicit in this conversation is the notion that the girl may have behaved "badly" because people around her failed in their responsibility to properly guide her. Giving advice is thus a duty for those who hold important knowledge and who are in the position to impart that knowledge. Consequently, once advice is given, it becomes the responsibility of the receiver to follow it—to modify their course. Thus risk avoidance is an individual's responsibility within the framework of an enabling social network.

When a woman has proved to herself that her husband is moving around with another woman, she may go to a female in-law for advice according to the idealized sequence of complain, confront, and send the spouse for counseling. Jessie Kwenda told us the steps one should take when confronting infidelity, saying, "Whenever faced with these problems, the first step would be to talk to him, and if that fails then third parties are involved, those could be his parents or aunties." According to Shupie Munthali, one must keep problems at home a secret until you reach a point where you can no longer endure. Only then do you consult a mother-in-law or father-in-law.

Some elders were confident in their ability to counsel couples through problems. Love Zgambo went to see her niece at home because her niece's husband was a womanizer. She counseled them and now claims that they are *kukhala makola*, that is, staying well. Below is an excerpt from our interview with Mrs. Zgambo:

> *R*: I told him these movements are not good [Mmm] because if you continue you will make your wife die and yourself.
> *I*: Eee – the disease?
> *R*: From the disease – so you need to abstain... He said what my wife told you was true so as you have advised me from today I will not continue. So I went to check on them [and they are staying well.]

Some women, such as Kettie Harawa, mentioned earlier for spying on her husband in the bushes, were fairly satisfied with the results of elder counseling. She reported to his grandmother that her husband was cheating, the grandmother intervened, and "now he has changed." Naomi Msiska was also happy with the help she received from her in-laws. When she married her current husband, she brought with her three children from a previous marriage. Her new husband changed his mind about marrying someone with so many children and decided to send her home. She reported to her in-laws. The elders told her husband, "You already knew about the children before you married; you should keep her." He did, and Naomi was happy with the intervention.

Not all women are so happy with their interventions. Masozi Nyirenda complained to her in-laws that her husband was not providing any money for *ndiwo*[18] for herself and the children. His parents criticized him, telling him that for the wife to remain respectable (one who is not begging around the compound or having boyfriends) you must give her money. Mr. Nyirenda apologized and said he did not know what he was doing and he would change his behavior. However, when we visited her for the third time, she was again troubled by beatings, his drunkenness, and lack of money. "Did you not say his behavior has changed?" we asked. She replied that his behavior changes when he has no money. As of now, she said, he is not communicating with his parents and they have given up on counseling him.

Competing Orthodoxies

The perceived lack of behavior change can cause despair, as demonstrated above, but can prompt some elders to encourage divorce and other unorthodox measures. Magret Kaonga, a middle-aged woman, tells the young women in her compound that if they suspect their husbands are HIV positive then they should get a blood test. If the blood test is positive then they should refuse to have sex with him. Elder Flora Kaonga counsels young women to begin having sex again earlier than the two-to-three year period traditionally recommended for postpartum abstinence, a period in which sex is considered dangerous and harmful to the nursing child. Flora, like many others, is concerned that men will go to other women during postpartum abstinence (Zulu, 2001), so to protect both the marriage and the child, she recommends ending abstinence early and using condoms to protect the child from danger. The use of condoms (especially by a married couple) and the ending of abstinence early are both practical innovations, because neither practice has high sociocultural value. Yet together they constitute an emerging unorthodox practice to secure fidelity.

Kettie Harawa, a twenty-year-old newlywed, was pregnant with her first child when we interviewed her. She said she could start having sex again after her child was six months old if she used condoms. Catherine reacted by laughing in shock and saying, "Which *agogo* supported condoms—the way *agogo* refuse condoms?" Catherine's shock demonstrates the novelty of an elder embracing the technology of condoms. Although there is a lot of talk about condoms in Malawi many people deem condoms problematic for a host of reasons; there are religious objections, concerns that condoms are ineffective or actually increase transmission of AIDS, and that they deaden pleasure. Alongside these objections is a concern that condom use signals a certain type of sexual relationship—not a trusting, exclusive and long-term relationship, but a sexual relationship involving a commercial sex worker and a client (Chimbiri, 2007: 1104). Thus condoms are seen as inappropriate in marriage. Kettie's casual acceptance of the advice suggests the power of elders to normalize a strategy through their authoritative recommendations. It should also be noted that a major campaign to promote the use of condoms for HIV prevention was launched in 1994 as Kettie and her agemates were coming of age. I suggest that though Kettie may have been more comfortable with the idea of condom use than the generations before her simply because of the times in which she was raised, the reinforcement by her elder advisor helped to frame condom use in marriage as both proper and good.

The influence of elders in defining what constitutes proper sexual behavior bears further investigation. When a woman moves into the marital village, the female elders from her family as well as her husband's family come with supplies and advice. On these occasions women learn from their elders that sex is a way to take care of a husband. The women told us that they were taught how to "dance" or "wiggle the hips" to help their husbands reach a climax. Some aunts would simulate sex for the couple to observe and learn, while others would instruct while having the couple simulate sex themselves. Though sometimes Tumbuka girls were trained by elders to "dance" before becoming engaged, they were not told the reason. Upon marriage women were also taught to clean the genitals of themselves and their husbands' after sexual intercourse, change and wash the bedclothes, and prepare "tea" (black tea and a snack of bread, groundnuts, or whatever small food is available) for the husbands to eat to renew their strength. Throughout the early days of marriage, women consult elders for advice on marital issues, including sex and child spacing. Elders are thus quite active in defining and supporting "proper" or "normal" sexuality for the younger generation.

The active role of elders in the sex lives of younger men and women is common throughout sub-Saharan Africa and initiations are important contexts through which sexual mores and norms are communicated. In Malawi, initiations dramatize the belief that the sex lives of individuals are intimately intertwined with the health of the village as a whole. During puberty, maturity, and marriage rites, youth are taught when and with whom it is proper to engage in sexual intercourse and when to abstain. They are instructed not to violate sexual taboos or risk bringing about *mdulo* illness to a third party. In his treatise on Chewa religion, van Breugel defines *mdulo* (also know as *tsempho* and related to subcategories of *kanyera* illnesses brought on by moral infringement) as taboos related to sexual activity. More specifically, *mdulo* is an illness complex related to the designation of certain sexual activities and bodily fluids (menstrual blood, sperm) as either "hot" or "cold." Old people, children, and people who have abstained from sex for a long time are considered relatively "cool." Sperm and menstrual blood are considered hot and it is dangerous to mix hot and cold in certain ways. Sexual intercourse is considered a hot state. Thus women who are breast-feeding are not supposed to also be having sex as the "hot" nature of her sexual activity can endanger the "cool" nursing child. van Breugel observed that when a woman had difficulty giving birth the older women attending her would urge her to confess adultery as it was believed that mixing the "blood" (sperm) of different men had brought about the problem. If the woman maintained her innocence, her husband was confronted for having committed adultery. If the wife died in childbirth, he was declared to be guilty of adultery (van Breugel, 2001: 178).

Mdulo taboos are many, various, and complex, impacting a wide array of daily activities because of their spiritual and familial dimensions.

> As one informant commented: "In order to make us follow this law our ancestors threatened us with this dreadful thing. If you commit adultery, your child will die, a pregnant woman will die in child-birth. Moreover Chauta [God] will be angry, your cattle will die, wild

> animals and diseases will not leave the village. All this they say to make us follow the law forbidding adultery." (van Breugel, 2001: 170–171)

While some (e.g., Marwick (1965)) saw *mdulo* as impersonal and non-spiritual in nature because the punishments for violating *mdulo* taboos come automatically, van Breugel informants all made connections between punishment and the authority of ancestors. In inculcating youth with *mdulo* norms and advising them with respect to proper sexual relations, elders are not perceived as simply indulging their own whims, but upholding the authority of ancestors and promoting the health of the community as a whole. By drawing on the authority of ancestors and seeking to protect the community from the displeasure of those ancestors the counsel of elders is endowed with added weight. Tensions arise when youth are seen as ignoring the advice of elders.

Several studies show that while tensions between generations have always existed, the focus of those tensions changes focus over time. In the AIDS era, some elders accuse the youth of an increasing lack of discipline and refusal to listen to them; they suggest that growing sexual promiscuity is the cause of the epidemic (Kaler, 2001; Kerr et al., 2008; Peters, Kambewa, and Walker, 2010; Schoffeleers, 1999). In Kaler's study in Southern Malawi, elder informants complained that youth no longer respected their wisdom, lack sexual discipline and restraint, had too many partners, were not afraid of death (AIDS), married and divorced on whims, did not follow child-spacing advice, married without proper procedures, and made decisions without consulting them. Kaler categorized the underlying concerns in these complaints into two types: complaints of atomization and of ephemerality. Marriages were seen as ephemeral—fragile, fleeting, and built on a whim. Marriages were seen as being built without the involvement of a wide circle of extended family input and involvement—atomization. The perception that unstable marriages were new to the younger generation did not bear out in research. In earlier periods (in Kaler example the 1940s), there were also high divorce rates and serial matrimony. There was also a tendency to see the youth as rebellious against elders. According to Kaler, her informants were carrying on a tradition of seeing marriages as fragile and in crisis but they failed to see that unstable marriages were not a new phenomenon but long a part of marriage in Southern Malawi (Kaler, 2001). Indeed, just as elders overestimate the newness of marriage crises, they may be simultaneously underestimating their own influence.

Despite the grumbling of some elders they probably yield more influence than they realize. In an article entitled "We Grandmothers Know Plenty" by Kerr et al., the authors explore the roles of grandmothers of Northern Malawi in influencing the child feeding practices of younger women, especially daughters-in-law (2008).

> According to interviews, focus groups and observations, grandmothers are considered to be important sources of knowledge and advice in many arenas of life. They often live next door to a married couple, provide seed to the couple when they first get married, and provide advice on pregnancy and care of young children. Grandmothers pass information about child nutrition to other older women. Mothers have considerable influence over their sons' marital relationship. If a mother felt it necessary, she could recommend divorce for her sons. A mother-in-law could take away a child from a mother if she felt the child was not being cared for properly. (2008: 1100)

Elders who give advice are seen as authorities to younger women in their accumulation of wisdom and knowledge and also because they have the ability to enforce consequences on women whom they feel are going astray in some way.

In scrutinizing interview transcripts, I discovered that the type of advice a person is likely to receive is far more associated with the particular role of the advisor within the kinship system than I had anticipated. Before I began the writing process, I drew out of the transcripts an assortment of women's strategies and was surprised to find that more than a few young women had been told by elders to divorce or go home to their natal village if there was unbearable trouble in the marriage. On closer inspection, I came to see that only elders from the natal village and some agemate friends were suggesting this type of action. Likewise, advice to use love medicines seemed quite common, but no one had been told to use these medicines by elder in-laws.

"Love Me" Medicine

The use of love medicine in Malawi is hardly new. Both men and women have long used love medicines in Malawi and throughout the region (Barnes, 1951; Kaler, 2001; Mitchell, 1951). What is new is the use of love medicine in the context of the AIDS epidemic. Shona and Ndebele women of Zimbabwe use "husband-taming herbs" as part of everyday practices for preventing their husbands from such undesirable behaviors as excessive drinking, gambling, and infidelity. These women explicitly see their usage of husband-taming herbs as a way to avoid contracting AIDS. The same holds true in Malawi. In my research one theme that arose again and again in stories of women's use of love medicine (called *temwanani*, "love one another" in Chitumbuka or *konda ine*, "love me" in Chichewa) is concern with men's mobility.

While both men and women can be accused of being "movious," that is, prone to the sexual mobility of having multiple partners, men are expected to be mobile in multiple ways. They are expected to seek work outside the home—maybe in nearby town, one of Malawi's cities, or farther afield in another country. Yet, as Kaler points out, mobility and travel are potent symbols of HIV (2003). Indeed, 13,000 Malawian migrant laborers working South Africa between 1988 and 1992 the South African Chamber of Mines were repatriated to Malawi. They Chamber of Mines claimed that the Malawians were responsible for the spread of HIV in South Africa. The concern with the link between HIV and labor-related mobility is offset by a desire of all parties concerned to enjoy the benefits of wage labor and cash income. "By all parties involved" I refer, not simply to husbands and wives but to their extended families as well.

Popular stories circulate of men who, using special medicines (*chithumwa*, singular and *vithumwa*, plural) from healers, travel far distances in the blink of an eye, enabling them to work in lands far away while maintaining a relationship with their wives and families. In some of these tales, the wife of a long absent husband becomes pregnant and is accused by her in-laws of sleeping with someone other than her husband (Wilson, 2012). To prove her innocence, the wife meddles with her husband's charms so that he is unable to return to his far away work site after one of his nightly visits. When morning comes the husband is still at his home and his relatives see he is really there. Because he is unable to go back to his job far away he angrily inquires of his wife "What have you done?" Such stories can be seen as an apologetic for women who find new lovers while their husbands are away, but they also highlight the stress imposed on families from migrant labor. In Malawi, migrant labor is gendered and it is men who are most likely to participate. This movement is welcome by the family of the man as well as his wife but poses problems for both.

Wives are often concerned that men will be spending time with other women, either commercial sex workers or women who could potentially be long-term girlfriends or wives. These women and the delights of the city could draw a man away from his loyalties at home. A man's natal kin may be concerned that the man's loyalty is divided both by the temptations of the city and his wife. Popular stories are rife with these conflicting concerns and allegiances. The migrant workers themselves also express fear about becoming detached from their homelands and families.

The selfsame traveling charms, *vithumwa*, men use to travel great distances also keep them tethered to their families on a spiritual realm. Generally speaking, *vithumwa* are used by laborers to deal with the insecurity of travel, employment, and economic advancement. The medicines are usually obtained from a healer in the area of their origin. Men keep possession of them or else they not only endanger the success of their economic endeavors but also endanger the very lives of their families. Indeed, one journaler reported a story wherein his neighbor had to return from South Africa because he had lost his *chithumwa* while he was drinking at a bar. Having become drunk the man got into a fight and the medicines (which are enclosed in a pouch) were removed from his underwear where they'd been sewn for safe keeping. He was called home the next day because of the death of his son (Wilson, 2012).

While wives desire the economic gains that may be made by a man's migration and his use of *vithumwa*, they are sometimes uneasy with the tradeoff. Another journaler reported the story of a woman who was jealous of her husband's new town wife. After the husband visited she took his *vithumwa* and threw it in the toilet. When the husband discovered he asked if she wanted him to die, saying that without the *vithumwa* he would have no way of "doing business and getting money" (Makombe MDICP journaler, August 2009).

Another woman lamented the loss of her husband to his new wife in town and all the consequences that accompanied that loss:

> Is it true that my husband has divorced me because he has married a Yao woman? I was used to sleeping with a man at night and I was working with him at the garden. Now what he has done will not help me. I will be feeling loneliness and I will be working alone in my garden. Will I be harvesting as I was doing with him? I am afraid because he will come to take his *Chithumwa* (Small pillow covered with herbs inside). He will come to take it out from my garden which means that

> I will not be harvesting more maize as I was doing with him. I will summon him so that he should tell me why he is leaving me. (Alice MDICP journaler, June 2009)

The woman was lamenting the loss of companionship, sex, and the removal of the husband's economic contribution. Her rival in the city was said to have used her own powerful medicines to draw the husband away, love medicine.

Many of the women I interviewed in 2006 had either used love medicine themselves or knew of a friend who used them. Love medicine was a clever answer to the conundrum of trying to affect a spouses' behavior without having to do so with an open confrontation. Women, in control of the cooking, could secret the medicine into food. Other medicines are sought to cause a man to lose desire for another partner or lose the ability to perform sexually with another partner. Men and women could even get medicine to "lock" one another sexually (Wilson, 2012). One woman, Ruth, told us she hid the medicine under a pillow so that her husband would in his sleep reveal the name of his lover. Some swear by the remedy and/or combine it with other approached to infidelity prevention. One journaler reported this conversation between several men about love potions:

> He said that other [some] wives go to a traditional doctor and get medicine and he said that traditional doctors most of the times advise them to put the medicine in the food that she prepared for the husband and once the husband ate the food he always simply follow the wife's command and the husband can do some pieces of work which could be done by a wife, such works include, cooking, cleaning plates, washing clothes, fetching water even bathing the children.
>
> Then another one said that the medicine is called "*Konda Ine*" in Chichewa and in English it means "love me" and other medicine are called "*Zungulira Khonde*" and others call it "*Mawazo*." This medicine makes the man to stay at the house most of the time since the husband was not staying at the house. If he used to drink beer at a bar or around the village he starts asking the wife to buy beer and drink at the house.
>
> His friends said that these medicines are not good sometimes they can make the husband become mad and sometimes the husband can become an idiot which will need much care from the wife and sometimes the husband can die due to the power of the medicine. But most of the times those women who use the medicine come up with good results only few have bad results. (Patuma MDICP journal, July 2004)

Though seen as generally efficacious, love medicines are described as causing a kind of madness—in particular, a madness of male feminization (doing women's chores) and emasculation (failure to do male work outside the domestic realm). Indeed, if the love medicines worked too well they caused a man to love his wife "too much," become "dormant," and get trapped in the domestic realm, no longer providing the economic support to the wife or family. Yet the alternative of not using love medicine is that one could perhaps lose her husband to the city and city women.

A man's kin are also concerned with the use of love medicine and the risk of a man loving his wife "too much." This, no doubt, accounts for the differences in who suggests love medicine to whom. The women I spoke to were advised to use love potions by their own relatives back home rather than from the elders in their husbands' villages. The elders among a woman's affinal relatives do not want her husband to be "too loving" of their wives:

> He continued saying that a lot of husbands are failing to assist their relatives as well as parents due to the reason than their wives gave them "*konda ine*" that whenever the woman rather the wife doesn't allow him to go to see and help this relatives mother or father then the man doesn't go but going unless [only] to see relatives . . . unless she allows him to go. (Simon MDICP journal, December 2004)

A fundamental tension seems to exist between a desire to promote male mobility and the desire to keep men tethered to home. Cautionary tales warn women away from taking the risk of immobilizing their husbands, but for women in the AIDS era it may well be better than the alternative—that is for a husband to bring home HIV. One woman told her friend that after some time being married her husband's behavior changed so that he did not love her anymore. She consulted with a traditional doctor in fear of her life:

> She told the other ladies what she has seen before happening to other women around by not [being] concerned with their husband's behaviours, which in turn brought them AIDS. The woman who collected the charms only asked for proper advice from her friends on the problem. (Chibwana MDICP journal, August 2005)

While much of the counsel given by natal kin overlaps with what affinal kin advice, some strategies suggested diverge from that given by affinal kin. This is true for love medicines and is also true in women's accounts of divorce, or "going home." This next section explores how women draw strength from their natal home in negotiations within marriage and as an ultimate refuge.

Divorce

When women fail to control the behavior of their husbands, some of them divorce. An elderly woman and second wife to the headman told us in an interview that complaints about AIDS are so common now that they are like a "song." When she hears about women in danger, she advises them first to counsel the husband and, if that fails, to go home. When problems arise,

> *R*: Just discuss with him... [warning him that] now there is AIDS. He will infect you and you will die. So if you have children they will be orphans. If he does not listen just leave him there—when he has contracted AIDS.
>
> *I*: And you go back?
>
> *R*: Yes
>
> *I*: Should leave him there?
>
> *R*: Should leave him there alone with his diseases. He will live here, go to Phukwa [town] and contract the disease and should infect me?! If he is known just leave him. (Chipeta, January 2006)

The complaints of women are like a refrain. Recall the folktale in which the woman stranded in her husband's village is rescued by her song that reveals her plight and results in her rescue and eventual return to natal kin. The girl cannot rescue herself but relies upon others to become extricated from possible consumption and destruction by her husband and affines. A woman's wariness of in-laws expressed in the tale resonates with a pattern I discerned in the predominant source of advice to "come home."

Advice to go home was given primarily to girls raised in the village and marrying out rather than to young women who were marrying into the village. Agness Kumwenda counsels new brides leaving the village to live with their new husbands to first discuss problems with the husband, and if that fails, go home to parents. My understanding that bridewealth makes parents reluctant to encourage divorce of their daughters was overset by the testimony of young wives. There was a surprising willingness on the part of some elders to support or even encourage divorce. Tawonga Chihana told us that before she was married, her aunts said that if a man is cheating on you you should come straight home because of this disease. The elders instructed that, if necessary, she should write a letter and they would come and bring her home. Her sister actually did this, she said. Witness Ngwira, a wife in her early twenties, was given similar advice. If the husband does not stop going with girlfriends after counsel then go straight home—he can kill you. Most of the young women knew of at least one friend who had left a husband because of infidelity. Some of the women had done so themselves, though it is unclear as to whether "going home" is always equivalent to divorce.

When Pauline Nyirongo, a woman in her twenties, confronted her husband over his infidelity, he beat her. She did not bother to report him for counseling at his village but went straight home. Her family welcomed her there, she said. For Pauline and her husband Simon, the separation was not permanent. Sometimes a separation initiates a divorce while at other times it initiates a reconciliation on the wife's natal territory. In Pauline's case, Simon followed her to the village and apologized to both her and her family. She decided to return to their marital home. We asked Pauline what her parents said to her husband to resolve the problem. She said,

> *R*: They forgave him because it was the first time. They said to him never to do it again. 'If a woman is wrong we don't beat, we just talk,' they advised him.
>
> *I*: What about the issue of sleeping at Phukwa [in town with other women], because here you have spoken about the beating issue only?
>
> *R*: They advised him it is not good to sleep out if you are married.

Why would Pauline bypass the counsel of her elder in-laws? One possibility is that she feared that these relations would not be able to bring about a satisfying resolution. In examples presented earlier in this chapter, we saw that interventions of in-laws could be frustrating for young women. Perhaps by seeking aid at home Pauline, and others, are able to negotiate marital conflicts from a position of greater strength. Parents and other elders related to a woman may be more likely to take a harsher stance against the husband's behavior than his own relatives. In Pauline's natal compound, Simon is surrounded by his in-laws rather than his own relations. The threat of a permanent separation is made more real by a woman's trip home and a confrontation with the people who can help make a separation permanent.

A woman's maintenance of connection with her natal home appears to play an ongoing role in her protection. When Vera Msukwa from the northern most District of Malawi received a proposal from a man from Karonga, her relatives were apprehensive. They warned her not to marry so far from home. From a distance it would not be easy for her to call upon her relatives when she was in need. In the case of Witness Ngwira, her natal relatives did not want her to marry so young, so they refused to accept bridewealth and other wedding fees from her husband's family. They wanted to be able to sever the marriage with few complications should problems arise. In some of the cases of going home or divorce reported to us, the natal kin welcomed their children home and in a few reported cases the natal kin went so far as to fetch the beleaguered wife and bring her home.

Like the folktale introduced early in this chapter, the natal home is the only safe haven for a wife troubled by her husband and in-laws. A woman's status as a stranger in her husband's village, though mitigated by time and the birth of children, may extend for many years. If a woman finds it too dangerous or disagreeable to remain married, she may leave and never return to her marriage by going home and sometimes by remarrying immediately. Several studies of virilocal societies have shown that natal kin can act as a strong support system even after a woman's marriage ends (Deluz, 1987; Hakansson, 1994; Kuper, 1958; Fricke et al.1993; Ngubane, 1987; Niraula and Morgan, 1996; Warner, 2007).

Fear of a bride entering into a vulnerable position vis-à-vis her husband and in-laws is found the world over sometimes expressed in the rituals of the weddings themselves. In primarily patrilocal Romania, Gail Kligman found that the wedding was an act that incorporates a bride into a position subordinate to her elder female in-laws (1984: 170). A daughter-in-law was expected to work hard, obey her mother-in-law, and to behave in a sexually honorable way (1984: 170). The wedding in Romania dramatizes the separation of a woman from her natal family such that the symbolism of the wedding is tied to idea of the bride's death.

By contrast Blake states that Chinese weddings are free of all reference to death to emphasize sexual maturation, fertility, and life. The exception, however, is in the practice of the bride's laments, which start three days before the wedding. In these mournful laments a bride weeps her farewells to her family, rebukes her parents for their matchmaking, and mourns difficulties to come. Blake quotes Yang Pi-Wang, who collected bridal laments in the hinterlands of Shanghai. Yang said, " 'The daughter fearing maltreatment by her in-laws and stern rule of her husband would be reluctant to leave her home' "(Blake, 1978: 15). Similarly the nuptial poetry of Estonia expresses the anxieties of a woman going into the strange territory of her husband's home (S. 1885: 169).

The Tumbuka of Northern Malawi at one time followed a matrilineal, uxorical local pattern of marriage common to Central African peoples. However, in the mid-nineteenth century Ngoni peoples traveled up from the Southern tip of Lake Tanganyika and conquered the Tumbuka (Kishindo, 2002). The result was a profound shift in language for the Ngoni and marriage practices for the Tumbuka. As the Tumbuka practices shifted toward the use of bridewealth marriages, patrilinearity, and virilocality, so rituals surrounding marriage also shifted. Young observed that a new etiquette arose in which "the new wife at her husband's village, affected uncontrollable grief and refused to touch food at all" once installed in her marital village. The mother-in-law exhibited alarm and offered food and beads to the young woman who would nibble on the food. This process was repeated until the coming of a group of girls from the village of the bride. They would finish the scraps of food left by the wife and later the husband would come forward with a gift of a hoe or beads. These gifts and the acceptance of them by the wife signaled the wife's acceptance of her wifely duties—productive, reproductive, and sexual. While Young focuses his interpretation of the issues of bridewealth and exchange (Young, 1931: 86–87), another reading of this dramatization would be that the tears and refusal to eat signify the anticipation of the difficulties of separating from ones' relatives to live among strangers. The concerns expressed by this scenario continue to trouble Tumbuka brides today.

The potentially contentious situation of a marital home is in some situations mitigated by a bride's continuing relationship with her natal family. In the context of patrilineal societies of sub-Saharan Africa, brothers in particular are described as being bound to sisters by the payment of bridewealth to the family. The receipt of cattle bridewealth for a sister's marriage makes a brother's marriage, and thus the continuance of the linage, possible. Wives, particularly in the early years of marriage, will live a life divided between their natal and affinal kin by making visits home to help to cultivate the fields or attending funerals. Women, therefore, maintain status in their home villages and call upon their families for assistance when necessary, receiving financial aid, marital advice, and a place to stay when problems arise (Deluz, 1987; Hakansson, 1994; Ngubane, 1987).

Discussion

Secrets hidden in dark places are illuminated by words. Malawian women place high value upon information that can shed light on the nature and behavior of the men they marry. The expectation that a man will change after marriage makes information gathering vital even after the wedding. Yet because they are "strangers," with their positions in their new homes precarious, younger women may feel themselves more vulnerable to deception or lacking in support. They turn to elders to guide the way through marital conflict, some finding the help they seek, while others look to agemates or elders from home. While it is generally accepted by the women I interviewed (with a few exceptions) that "marriage is endurance," what that means varies. For some, endurance had the meaning of passive resignation to infidelity or other difficulties. For others still, endurance had more of a sense of perseverance and active intervention.

The model of the individual or even of a couple making decisions about their sexuality is at odds with the reality of many Malawians. Elders and other family members are very involved in the decision-making processes relating to sex and reproduction in marriages. This is hardly a new insight about family structures and functioning in the region. Thus the prevailing public health AIDS messages and education crafted around the notion of individual decision making fall not on deaf ears but on ears listening to many tunes. An alternative approach would be to ensure that not only can women and men consider their risk and options but also they can be supported in their decisions by people in their social network who have influence and authority in their lives. Tapping into local stakeholders to promote health should not mean simply bringing a chief, village head, or religious leader on board, but mobilizing a greater preexisting network of elders and authorities in their informal and familial capacities to support sexual and reproductive health of younger generations (Kerr et al., 2008; Muturi and Mwangi, 2011).

Seeking advice from elders, confronting a spouse, and meeting as a couple for counseling with an elder were the standard first steps for resolving conflict. The strength of such interventions is that they are made through people in the community who can impose sanctions, that is, elders. Some women we spoke to felt their problems with a husband's infidelity were solved by elder intervention. This was not the case for everyone, however. Other women found it necessary to take advice from different sources and looked to friends and natal kin to provide them with solutions that in-laws would rarely suggest—love potions and divorce are among these. Some actions taken by women are not likely to be promoted by advisors. Chapter 3 explores strategies of aggression wherein women attack the women that are objects of their husbands' attention.

CHAPTER 3

FUNNY, YET SORROWFUL: NARRATIVES OF EMPOWERMENT AND EMPATHY IN WOMAN AGAINST WOMAN STRUGGLES

Introduction

As in many places around the world, in Malawi stories about marital conflicts and sex scandals provide engaging and entertaining topics of conversation. Despite the universality of the topic, however, these stories are shaped by locally and regionally distinctive concerns, plot structures, imagery, and motifs. Indeed, some stories may be said to fall into patterned narrative genres. Such is the case with accounts in Malawi of a woman fighting another woman about a man with whom both claim a sexually intimate relationship. The woman against woman fight story genre provides a framework not only for recounting such struggles but also for interpreting them. In this chapter, I present narratives of wives challenging sexual rivals as a way to explore the logic and impact of woman against woman aggressive strategies, and also interrogate the role that oral narratives play in these dramas.

Aggression can take several forms and be used for multiple reasons. In their efforts to ensure fidelity of their spouses, women in rural Malawi may resort to aggressive or confrontational strategies that challenge female rivals, that is, the "other" woman in their husbands' lives. These challenges can take the form of physical aggression or social aggression. Physical aggression involves a bodily attack on another person or their property, while social aggression involves persuasion or marshaling opinion against a rival in a community. The aim of either type is to force the "other woman" away from the contested husband and from the village if possible, that is, expulsion. Mary Douglas calls such tactics "strategies of exclusion" (Douglas, 1991). Women may resort to aggression when other tactics for influencing the fidelity of their spouses fail. Aggressive tactics are also used when women wish to avoid uncomfortable or dangerous confrontations with husbands.

Gossip and fight narratives play an important role in strategies of exclusion. My analysis of fight narratives highlight the centrality of labeling rivals in both physical and social aggression strategies. People who slander and label sexual rivals through rumor and gossip often stigmatize their opponents as threats to the health of the community. Labeling someone as an outsider, trouble maker, prostitute, or AIDS widow is a weapon in a woman's arsenal against another woman. The power of some of these labels is intensified by the discourse of vulnerable populations and at risk groups perpetuated through AIDS public health campaigns. AIDS education campaigns in Malawi and throughout Southern and Eastern Africa identified sex workers, mobile populations, and widows as highly at risk groups. The effect of these campaigns is that "at risk" and "vulnerable" groups are not only perceived by the public as in need of support and intervention but are also perceived as dangerous and culpable. Women who want to exclude other women from the lives of their husbands may attempt to affix the "at risk" label to a rival to marginalize her as a dangerous outsider. Indeed, there has been a great deal of anxiety surrounding practices of AIDS stigmatization expressed by scholars and public health officials. However, my research reveals that seldom is the outsider or marginal identity of a rival firmly fixed within a community. The stories told about woman against woman fights make explicit the tentative nature of labeling and the tenuous status of the women who try to employ labels. Indeed, these stories are characterized by a great deal of ambivalence; they explore women's sources of strength and vulnerability, they are stories of triumph and sadness. Malawians describe tales of infidelity and aggressive confrontation as highly entertaining and yet simultaneously sad or shameful. Ultimately these fight stories suggest that woman against woman confrontations are at once a kind of collective catharsis of scapegoating and a shameful or morally questionable opposition of vulnerable woman against vulnerable woman.

I Caught Him with An/"other" Woman

My first introduction to woman against woman fight narratives took place back in 2003 when I was introduced to hundreds of Malawi Diffusion and Ideational Change Project (MDICP) ethnographic journals. These journals are reports of conversations written by Malawians who worked as interviewers for the MDICP, a longitudinal study of beliefs and practices relating to sexuality, AIDS, and marriage. The journals, commissioned by the project to supplement the quantitative data being collected, contain a rich array of narratives about sexuality and AIDS. Accounts of sexual rivals committing violence against one another stood out as a distinctive genre. In the narrative presented below many of the features of the genre are apparent. One young woman told a journaler about her skirmish with her husband's girlfriend and the dramatic events leading up to the conflagration. The journaler, a young man in his 20s, wrote

> We laughed. She continued, "I caught him with another woman, moreover our neighbor...doing sexual intercourse in my house [in the] afternoon when I went to the market and returned fast because I didn't fulfill my appointments I scheduled that day as he thought I will be late with those appointments. He asked the partner to visit him in the afternoon, so she did and the woman was as well married and [that] marriage ended the same day as well. I found them totally doing sex at my bedroom and I was furious that I caught the woman at the neck and we started fighting and she was losing and the husband kept on holding me so that I may not be able to fight her thoroughly as I was intending to. Then neighbors came to rescue us and then neighbors criticized the woman and she felt very shamed. In the following day morning I departed coming here while he went in town say to shop maternity goods for me, I was not after that, I departed without him knowing..."
>
> And I [the journaler] asked why she did like that?
>
> [The journaler's] in-law said, "I wanted to give him the lesson that he may not repeat that, and make him know that I hated that."
>
> [The journaler's] wife said, "And if he comes you may allow him to be your husband once again?"
>
> In-law said, "Ooh! Yes, I will allow because our marriage didn't end but we have just separated because of what he did, and moreover I have his child who may need his assistance." (Bato, MDICP research journal, February 2002)

Like many narrations of sexual rivalries, the story contained standard elements including the revelation of infidelity (by chance or by design), a verbal and/or physical fight, an account of the spouse's actions (often either running away or protecting girlfriends), and a description of the reactions and interventions of neighbors. Finally narrators of fight narratives usually end with discussion of the consequences of the confrontation. In the excerpt above the wife discovered the infidelity accidentally and flew into a rage. The community reacted by intervening on behalf of the wife and imputing shame to the rival. Through the fight and the separation the woman sought to teach her husband a lesson.

It became clear after reading a dozen such stories that fighting between women is both a strategic and an emotional response to infidelity. In addition, it is often a response that relies upon collectivities. Sometimes neighbors and friends will join into the fight and become participants in a friend's struggle for fidelity.

The narrative presented above was set in Southern Malawi among the matrilineal and uxorilocal Yao, that is, in a context in which descent is traced through the female line and married couples typically live in the birth village of the wife. In such a context one might expect a relatively high level of such assertiveness because women there are surrounded by their own kin. However, even among the virilocal Tumbuka of Northern Malawi, where women leave their birth families to live among their husbands' families, this kind of narrative is quite common and remarkably similar to those told in the South. In the next journal excerpt from Northern Malawi, the journaler writes about a man who was caught having sex with a "young girl" (presumably a teenager). His wife and her friend caught the illicit couple and beat the girl. The women's retelling of the tale is full of laughter and self-congratulations, a common feature of these stories.

> Since there is no secret under the sun, one day Anderson went out to have sex in the bush with a certain young girl. [It was] funny but shame[ful] what happened... While they [were] having sex, a group of women came to that bush fetching for firewood. Unfortunately those women fetching for firewood went straight to where these two... were having sex as if they were told... where these guys were.... [A]mong them was a wife of the man (Anderson). They found these two... The... wife of Anderson was... very angry and the fighting started there. The husband (Anderson) ran and left the fighting

> on. The...women joined the fighting against the young girl. Though the husband ran but he didn't go far he was just hidden by the anthill. So he was watching what was happening to his girlfriend. He failed to control himself not to go stop the fighting. And his girlfriend was bloody [over] the whole body. And those women instead of fetching firewood they all joined fighting. So the husband came out from that behind anthill. You women, stop beating her, she is young she is not your age, hey my wife don't beat her. I have just [had] sex once with her. And if you are not stopping beating her then I will not leave her said the husband (Anderson). The husband came to the fight stopping them fighting. It took about 10 minutes to stop the fighting. By the time the fighting was over the girl was almost bloody, especially her face and chest.
>
> The other women who were with the wife of Anderson to fetch firewood started laughing at their friend (wife) of Anderson that without their help she (wife) would have been lost the fighting. They didn't even fetch the firewood...after the fighting. And they all went home laughing, reviewing what was happening when they were fighting. (Chipeta, MDICP research journal, September 2003)[1]

The laughter that characterizes this narrative is typical of one of several discernible patterns in women's fight narratives. The collective nature of the struggle is also a common feature. In the narratives presented above the conflict between a woman and her rival becomes the conflict of her friends as well. Often the husband flees the scene or protests from a distance, displaying his relative lack of power in that particular instance. Furthermore, fighting, though often erupting in moments of heated or unexpected confrontations, can be a part of a self-conscious strategy for a woman to gain control over her husband's fidelity. We saw this in the case where the woman says she was trying to teach her husband a lesson. However, fights do not emerge out of thin air. How are fights the unveiling or eruption of ongoing conflicts between rivals that on an everyday basis entail complaints, gossip, and labeling as primary exclusion tactics? What do they reveal about the nature of the conflict and the relative social influence of the sparring women? And finally, what kinds of success do women achieve and what role does humor and camaraderie play in constructing success? How does women's eruption into laughter signal a momentarily eruption of empowerment or agency? To answer these questions I draw upon Mary Douglas' theories relating to practices used to exclude individuals.

Strategies of Exclusion

The term "strategies of exclusion" is derived from the work of Mary Douglas and refers to the means by which a society marginalizes certain members (Douglas, 1991). In the article "Witchcraft and Leprosy," she lays out two strategies of rejection, both of which are based on accusations of insidious harm. For the purpose of this chapter we are most interested in her theory that societies use "infectious disease as a resource for controlling designated public enemies." The person being rejected need not start as a marginal figure but can become one in a process of negative accusations. Douglas names two factors necessary in successful strategies of rejection: "There has to be consensus. There has to be an imputation of immorality (724)."

The first step in excluding a rival is to affix to them a negative label, that is, to verbally or otherwise accuse them of belonging to a group to which society ascribes negative characteristics and behavior (Douglas, 1991: 725). The next step in rejection strategies is for an agent to put forth accusations of harm such that the accused is viewed as a threat to the public. In the context of Northern Malawi, and indeed much of sub-Saharan Africa the labels of "prostitute" and to a lesser extent "widow" fit the description of categories to which negative characteristics are attached. Both groups are considered part of AIDS "at risk" categories regularly targeted for public health campaigns and scholarly examination (Chirwa, 1997; Craddock, 2000; Hunt, 1989; Kishindo, 1995; Luginaah et al., 2005; Malungo, 2001; Mhalu et al., 1991; Okeyo and Allen, 1994; Schoepf, 2001; Waldby, 1996). While seen as "endangered" or vulnerable they are simultaneously viewed as potentially diseased and dangerous (Bird, 1996; Goldstein, 2004; Gould, 1993; Lawless, 1996; Sabatier, 1988).

It is here that I take a turn and resist going down the well-trod road of stigma scholarship. Issues of blame and discrimination have been well documented and analyzed (Lawless, 1996; Sabatier, 1988; Farmer, 1992; Treichler, 1999) as have the means by which stigmatized groups and individuals resist labels (Parker, 1987; Farmer, 1992; Schoepf, 1988) or make positive use of labels ascribed to them (Mutongi, 1999; Robins, 2006). Instead, I want to break away from this paradigm that has dominated medical anthropology and public health. The dominance of the paradigm has made thinking about strategies of exclusion in any other way seem impossible (Douglas, 1991: 734). By contrast,

I examine narratives about aggression and labeling from the perspective of women who seek to exclude "other" women from the lives of their husbands. By their efforts of exclusion women practice one of the avenues of agency open to them. Below I present five cases of woman against woman fights and evaluate the success of the strategies of exclusion from the perspective of the aggressors defending their marriages.

Mrs. Kuzunga versus the Prostitute

In a report written in February 2006 by rumor journaler Simon Nyirongo related a gory tale of adultery and violence involving a woman labeled as both "prostitute" and "foreigner/stranger." This narrative highlights the power of the labels of "prostitute" and "foreigner" to Northern Malawians. The association of prostitutes with AIDS is strong, as is distrust of foreigners or strangers. The fierceness of the beating received by the woman labeled as prostitute in this story may be related to the power of these labels and to the desire for collective protection from someone categorically reviled.

When Simon stopped by a clinic to collect money owed him by one woman, two other women entered and began to relate the scandalous story. In a Northern Malawian trading center, a woman named Mrs. Kuzunga heard rumors that her husband was sleeping with a prostitute while she was away at a funeral. When Mrs. Kuzunga arrived at her home she found her husband and the prostitute in bed, naked. Furious as "a hungry lion," according to the narrator, Mrs. Kuzunga grabbed a panga knife[2] and began to beat the woman with the knife. Meanwhile her husband fled the scene. When the prostitute got a chance, she also fled, bleeding from her hands and her head. Mrs. Kuzunga sent the houseboy to catch the woman.

The houseboy caught the woman, and Mrs. Kuzunga shouted for her friends. The neighbors crowded around and began questioning the "other woman." What did she think she was doing? Who was she? These neighbors presumed that she was a foreigner from Tanzania and a prostitute. The besieged woman told the crowd that Dr. Kuzunga had said he was a widower. She explained that they had been seeing each other for several years and that he promised to marry her. Someone in the crowd asked if the woman had used condoms. The woman replied that at first they used condoms but later the man insisted condoms were no longer necessary because of their faithfulness to one another.

This statement was a breaking point for Mrs. Kuzunga, according to the women relating the story to Simon Nyirongo:

> "Then as the prostitute was narrating Mrs. Kuzunga became very furious with the statements that the prostitute was narrating so she ordered the people who were around to play on her. So indeed the people started beating the prostitute. It was said that they were using different kinds of materials when they were beating the prostitute—materials such as panga knives, stones, sticks and some of the helpers used a razor blade which had left the prostitute big cut in the face, head, logs, arms, and a very big cut on her stomach."
>
> But the other source...said, "The mob even tampered with the private part of the prostitute with the aim of teaching her a lesson that it is bad to be making relationships the husbands of other people...the prostitute is not to be blamed for the shit that happened because it is Dr. Kuzunga who is very careless with her life. Of course the man is already aware that prostitutes are very dangerous people who do not care about their precious life, and that they are after money not love. And these prostitutes do not choose men, they just sleep with any man that comes on their way as long as the man has got cash at hand and it is believed that it is these prostitutes that are highly spreading the HIV/Aids to many people and in many countries usually because these people do sleep with lot of men whom they do not even know about their HIV status so in such a way there is a great chance of them get the HIV/Aids or spread it."
>
> The young lady kept on saying that she tends to wonder why some men [are] attracted to these prostitutes while they already know that sleeping with a prostitute is just the same as killing...yourself. (Nyirenda research journal, February 2006)

Although the prostitute is absolved of complete blame for the affair (e.g., "The young lady also said that the prostitute is not to be blamed for the shit that happened because it is Dr. Kuzunga who is very careless with her life"), nowhere in the conversation as related in the journal was there a sense that the violence inflicted upon the young woman's body was unwarranted and cruel. In fact, Mrs. Kuzunga appears as the heroine of the story. The act of violence can be interpreted as preventative and also as retributive. In this story retribution comes not only from Mrs. Kuzunga but also from her friends, who identify with their neighbor and friend and enter into the violence. Inasmuch as the prostitute—who remains nameless throughout—falls into the category of an "at risk" type, that is, sex worker, she comes to stand for all other prostitutes—all women who sleep with other people's husbands. The battered woman becomes a scapegoat, forced to take the punishment for other women. "The AIDS sufferer is a victim-turned-villain in the popular mind, recalling the lepers, and maimed, crippled evil-doers of popular culture" (Bird, 1996: 50).

Even so, assuming the narrative corresponds either to some real life events or is an exaggeration, why would these women react with such extreme violence? I suggest that the interpretation of the women's responses must be filtered through the lens of AIDS and uncertainty, or perhaps in this case, AIDS and certainty. In Simon's account of the beating, he consistently refers to the victim of the beating as "the prostitute." Her identity as a prostitute and a foreigner in the perception of the multiple narrators marks her as a dangerous, polluting other—a threat to the stability of marriages and community health. There is no trace of doubt in the assertions that the victim has HIV. She is a prostitute and foreigner, she is certain to have HIV. The magnitude of the response may be a function of the certainty of the belief and the extent to which the woman is an outsider.

By contrast, certainty about the HIV status of others seems to diminish as people trace outward from the types of people considered central to disease dissemination. Prostitutes are high on the list of those whom Malawians identify as sources of the disease. Though Dr. Kuzunga is considered at high risk of infection, more evidence is needed to confirm his diagnosis. The prostitute, however, is implicated through her identity as such, the husband's reputation as a womanizer needs to be established. The journaler reports a lengthy conversational exploration of Dr. Kuzunga's activities with prostitutes and school girls and his overall flirtatious behavior. People spoke even more doubtfully about the serostatus of the Kuzunga's wife (Nyirenda research journal, February 2006).

The site of greatest consensus was the body of the Tanzanian woman. Foreigner and "prostitute," she was utterly outsider, utterly "other." Her body was perceived as certainly diseased, and the community showed little pity or restraint in placing burdens of AIDS and infidelity on her shoulders and meting out punishment. She represented the embodiment of the diseased other, the threat to the wholeness of the community. One hopes, upon reading this account, that the violence has been grossly exaggerated. Even so, the extreme violence imagined in this narrative still constitutes a coalescence of public opinion and collective catharsis, a fantasy of revenge.

Furthermore, I also suggest that it was not only gossip and a slandered reputation that created the "other" woman's image of prostitute but also the public beating itself and the revealing of her genitalia that stabilized her label as prostitute. A conflict that could have remained private became a very public affair in which many people felt they had a stake. Her public shame became the proof of her guilt. In the end it is really public shame, rather than the physical beating per se, that was Mrs. Kuzunga's main weapon in the battle against her rival. In the next case, the identity of the "other" woman as outsider is less clearly defined.

Mrs. Kayira versus Eunice, the Spinster

One wife, Mrs. Kayira, targeted both the person and possessions of the new woman in her husband's life. In this case, the rival is described as a spinster, but she is firmly established in the community as a baker and long-time resident. Her position in the community, in fact, seems more firmly established than that of the wife. The relative social integration of Mrs. Kayira and her rival may have had more to contribute to the success or failure of the aggressive strategies than the violent actions themselves.

The journaler Hastings Mkandawire describes a conversation he had with Mrs. Gondwe when he visited with a message for one of the women of her house. Mrs. Gondwe, the main narrator, is a middle-aged divorcee. She lives with her mother Mrs. Mbale who is in her seventies. Mrs. Gondwe's daughter Mrs. Chavula is home for a visit. Mrs. Gondwe tells with relish the scandal of her neighbor Eunice, whom Hastings describes as a spinster.

> *I was warmly welcomed by the three ladies at the household [of] Mrs. Gondwe, Mrs. Chavula, and Mrs. Mbale. I got a small stool which was on the khonde*[3] *and [sat] on it. The thing I wondered [about] before I was greeted was [the] burning of the small house.*

> *Hastings*: Ah-ah, what happened to this small house here? You mean there was fire here the other time? Where was the lady when the house was catching fire? *This time Eunice was not at home she was at the Training Centre where she works as an assistant baker...*
>
> *Mrs.Mbale*: You know that we are keeping Eunice here in the house which [caught] fire last week. This girl started going out with

Mr. Chirwa who opened the Bar at Mphokwa Trading Centre. Understand the lady followed the money which that bar is making…

Hastings: Is Mr Chirwa not married?

Mrs.Gondwe: Ah, that man is older than my brother—he is married with three children. The wife and children do stay at home and he does stay here solely because of that bar business

Mrs.Chavula: If [he is] married why all these things? How can a person married indulge himself is boyish behavior?

Mrs.Mbale: My in-law, there are certain men who don't consider their age when doing things they always like to be young in needs…

Hastings: …What I want to know is what really happened to have the house catch fire?

Mrs.Mbale: Now, the wife of Mr. Kayira got the news from friend and the first action she took was to move from home where she was staying to Mphokwa T Centre to stay close to the husband. In other words guarding the husband from his careless behavior…

Mrs.Gondwe: Alongosi, alongosi mwapulika (*brother, brother, you heard). She always starts statements like that I then got attention to her. I know Mrs. Gondwe wanted to add something to the story.* That first move of coming to stay with the husband here didn't help the woman. We were seeing still Kayira coming to stay and even taking his night here.

Hastings: You mean he was leaving the wife alone at his house and coming to sleep with Eunice? So what was his own wife thinking over his missing in the house throughout the night?

Mrs.Mbale: Now it was her time to prove that what [she] was hearing from people—friends was really true. She came here one day to shout [at] the lady (Eunice) unfortunately Eunice was at work…she just kept her in mind.

Mrs.Gondwe: This was worsened when the wife of Kayira got the news that Kayira wants to marry Eunice. There was no peace at both sides—Sabela Kayira was in troubles at home same [as] was Eunice here. The woman was coming shouting at her. Out of all these efforts nothing was changing. As the result she just decided to kill a spinster by setting the house fire. She comes at very late hour around past one pm. The house was then set on fire. Eunice who was sleeping inside told us that she noticed smoke entering the house she wondered and quickly got out of the house while outside she wondered to see the roof under fire she shouted for help and her landlord, Mrs. Mbale and Mrs. Chawinga were the first to assist her keeping the[m] all out of fire. Water was used on that day to try to [put] out [the] fire. While we were doing this Gomezga who was the only man too [*sic*] come to assist us [was] busy inside to get the goods out of the house. When it was 3:00 pm the fire had stopped on the roof of the house. Now Mr. Gomezga wanted to know what caused [the] danger[ous] fire he went around to see if [the] fire might have started from ground grass [but] there was no trace of grass around the house... "Eunice, somebody have just set fire on your house roof or else the fire might have started inside the house and I quoted." She was Mrs. Chawinga who opened our eyes. She quickly reminded us of Sabela Kayira who has been coming to [the] house shouting at Eunice concerning their love affairs with Kayira.

Hastings: So she was the one responsible for the fires on the Eunice's house what followed after suspecting Sabela?

Mrs.Gondwe: The lady Sabela was in the following morning consulted on the story and the issue was taken to the village headman to answer some charges. Up to now we don't know what will follow after hearing the story from both parties. But the affairs between Kayira and Eunice are still going on.

In terms of content, the most striking difference between this text and that of the prostitute is that the "spinster" as adulteress is less clearly a villain than the prostitute of the previous story. Yes, she sleeps with another woman's husband, but she is not part of a recognized "at risk" group or portrayed as a risk to the community as a whole. She even seems poised to become a wife. Indeed, though she is called a "spinster" several times, primarily she is called by her name. She is integrated into the community and has an identity independent from her sexual activities in the account of the narrators. Recall that the narrators mention that Eunice works as an assistant baker at the bakery. According to Douglas Raybeck, the effect of multiple identities and a community's desire for reconciliation mitigate effects of labels, as stated below:

> If a person labeled as deviant remains a co-resident, other villagers seldom treat that individual in the dichotomous fashion suggested by Becker (1963), Matza (1969), and other labeling theorists. Instead, there is often recognition of and expressed value for other statuses the individual occupies, and continuing efforts are often made to reincorporate the individual into the mainstream of village life. (Raybeck, 1988: 387)

Even though Eunice's relationship to Mr. Kayira is comparable to the relationship the unnamed prostitute shared with Mr. Kuzunga, Eunice's actions were not judged with the same harshness. Some social theorists have suggested that it is not one's actions that define one as "deviant" but rather the willingness of a community to apply that label when an opportunity arises. "The deviant is one to whom that label has successfully been applied" (Becker, 1963: 9).

Eunice's integration, however, has dire impacts on Mrs. Kayira's ability to successfully attack and exclude her. Mrs. Kayira's fire, if she did indeed set it, did not succeed in scaring Eunice away. Instead, the act is described as a desperate maneuver in a losing battle. The women observed that the man continued to visit his girlfriend. The narrators also mentioned the failure of Mrs. Kayira's many other efforts to interrupt the relationship between her husband and Eunice. In this narrative, Mrs. Kayira is the outsider. She went outside her marital village, where she has perhaps developed a social support network, in order to challenge Eunice. She could not, therefore, call upon Eunice's neighbors to launch a public and shaming attack against her rival.

Instead she undertook a secretive attack to set a fire that brought the neighbors to the aid of Eunice instead of herself. Mrs. Kayira's secrecy can be interpreted as an indication of her lack of social support within that village and an admission of the shameful nature of her attack. I suggest that an open attack with the support of friends and neighbors implies righteous anger and retribution. In the end it is Mrs. Kayira's actions, more so than Eunice's that are called into question. Mrs. Kayira she does not enjoy the support of her peers within that village.

In contrast to the prostitute's tale, in this narrative shares of shame were more evenly distributed. The husband's "boyish" and impulsive behavior, Eunice's foolish but understandable "following money," and a desperate wife's violent attack all receive criticism in turn. Mrs. Kayira's failure to win the public battle to shame her rival stems both from her lack of integration in that particular context and Eunice's comparatively high level of integration. Part of Mrs. Kayira's failure was thus related to her own "outsider" status and to Eunice's advantage in the social terrain rather than "deviant" behavior per se.

Sabina and the Co-Wife

Even when a woman's confrontation with an "other" woman takes place in her marital village, she may find that she lacks support among key members of her affinal family network. Such was the case for Sabina Chirambo. Sabina and her in-laws had opposing views on whether her marriage should become polygamous. As a result, Sabina's effort to label her husband's girlfriend as dangerous and garner support in the village yielded limited success. When we asked Sabina about divorce cases she knew of relating to infidelity, and she said that she herself had divorced for that reason. "Divorce" is being loosely defined here and is not necessarily permanent. Sabina went home twice because of her husband's womanizing. She said she ran away because of diseases. She had gone to the elders in her marital village multiple times but she became tired of repeating this process. The aunts also became tired of advising her. Sabina confronted her husband and told him it was bad to womanize. "You will get the disease and you will not die alone, but it will kill both of us and our children will suffer" (March 7, 2006).

She first heard about her husband's womanizing from friends, and later the "other" woman came to stay in the village. We asked her to narrate her story. "What did she come to do? Why didn't you burn her?" Catherine asked while laughing. Sabina continued to knit while replying with a smirk, "She came to marry, A-a-a, can I just leave her [alone]?" Four months before our interview the woman had come to marry Sabina's husband Tobias. When the other woman first arrived in the village, Sabina was unaware because she was in her natal village at a funeral. Meanwhile, her husband was called before his elders because his girlfriend had arrived pregnant. They wanted him to accept the woman as his second wife. When Sabina arrived home from the funeral, she found her husband staying with the new wife at his grandmother's house.

Sabina's marital situation continued to deteriorate. Not only was Tobias now living in a house with the new wife but Sabina also could not find the money she had earned when she sold the tobacco. The money she planned to use for buying fertilizer was gone. She went after the "other" woman and beat her. She chuckled as she told us, "Yea, so my husband, [Mmm] my husband protected the new wife." The respondent, Catherine, and I laughed at the image of the scene and Catherine commented cannily, "*Vikusekeskanaso vyachitima.*" It is funny but also sorrowful. Is laughter an indication of classic "gallows humor" (Fine, 1988; Obrdlik, 1942)?

Folklorists, drawing on the work of Sigmund Freud (1960[1909]) and sociologist Obrdlik, have conceived of humor as a means to defend the psyche against dangerous or painful thoughts (Burke, 1989; Dundes and Hauschild, 1983; Fine, 1988). Fine has examined gallows humor as a means of collective buffering against a sense of overwhelming vulnerability to danger and uncertainty:

> Individuals and the communities they are part of may control this risk by continually talking about it... Fortunately, folklore genres, notably humor provide a means by which people can address their fear while convincing themselves that they are not afraid because they are able to joke about it. (Fine, 1988: 179)

Sabina's fear of infidelity is managed in her rehearsal of the fight narrative in which she is portrayed as assertive and in control of the immediate situation. The intervention of her husband is one more piece of evidence of her superior power and control. Key to this sense of control, according to Fine, are the personas that humorists embody when performing (1988: 177–178).

Fine's concept of persona is built upon Goffman's notion of "framing," in which a performance is marked off from the norm to be interpreted in a nonliteral "humor frame" that allows "comic license" such that everything within that frame is not to be taken seriously (Goffman, 1974). That is to say that the tendentious and possibly fractious opinion expressed within the humor frame is not to be attributed to the joker outside of that context. However, we find that Sabina's goal in framing and punctuating her story with humor and bravado has an opposing inclination. Sabina and other women who tell similar narratives desire for that persona of strength to be extended into their everyday image and persona. However, unlike classic "gallows humor" in which the joke is told from the perspective of the oppressed, Sabina's humor proceeds from a location of both strength and vulnerability. She demonstrates strength over her rival and her husband and perhaps even over her in-laws. However, her actions are in part derived from her position of weakness with respect to the wishes of her in-laws, husband, and the "other women." She is both the oppressed condemned of gallows humor and the hangman aggressor (Burke, 1989; Dundes and Hauschild, 1983), and the moment passes as one of humor and sorrow in which irreducible ambivalence is lodged. The fight and the moment of laughter were the high point of a narrative in which Sabina's strength was to be challenged again and again.

The initial fight precipitated a series of negotiations. Sabina threatened to leave, but her in-laws insisted that they all sit down together to settle the matter. Her husband claimed that he did not really love the new wife but that his aunt and grandmother were forcing him to take her. Sabina protested that this was a lie, because while she was away, he was freely with the woman. Eventually, however, husband and wife reconciled leaving the new wife alone at Tobias' grandmother's house. It seemed that Sabina's tactics had yielded some positive results. The husband was no longer staying with the new wife.

Later it was heard that the other woman began to go around with male tenant farmers. Sabina's husband went out of the district and while away heard that his second wife was sexually unfaithful. During that time Sabina was summoned before her in-laws. The grandmother and aunt told her that she was responsible for her husband refusing to accept the new wife. They threatened to call the police because of the beating if she did not leave, so Sabina she went to her parents' home. The environment had become too hostile. When Tobias returned, he found his first wife gone. Sabina reported, "Then that new wife was also chased away by my husband, and he said it's you, grandmother, who is keeping this wife. She is sleeping with tenants, she is a bargirl. Do you wish me good with my life?"

Tobias sent his new wife away and followed Sabina back to her home village. There, Sabina's parents refused to allow him to take her back. If you take her back, she can just die, they told him. They referred to AIDS. Her husband left but came back again with his own father to apologize and bring Sabina back to his village. Sabina returned to her marital home. "He has really changed," she said. Had Sabina "won"? Had she separated her husband from the "other" woman?

The story developed further. When we visited Sabina again she told us the other woman had been arrested for cheating people out of money. That seemed like victory for Sabina. By our third visit the cowife had returned to live in the village. We asked if the woman had recommenced her relationship with Tobias but Sabina was not certain. Sabina's triumph was fleeting and in some ways quite ignoble. Not only had she beat up a pregnant woman but had sent her to fend for herself. In the various versions of this story we heard from her neighbors, people said that the man refused to accept responsibility for his second wife. As the "other" woman gained the reputation of going out with tenant farmers, the magistrate did not take seriously the negligence suit she brought against Tobias. We are left to wonder what options are open to a woman thus rejected.

Sabina's story demonstrates the tenuous and temporary quality that a success can have when the "other" woman is not easily labeled and is accepted by key members of a community. In confronting her rival, Sabina was also confronting her in-laws, who actively sought to incorporate the new wife into the family. Unlike earlier cases where the "other" woman was identified as a prostitute throughout, the identity of the "other" woman here begins as a legitimate second wife who is pregnant and supported by her in-laws and welcomed by her husband. Sabina gains favor over her rival through her own machinations (i.e., the fight, the confrontation with her husband and in-laws, and the negotiations taking place at her natal home) and the new wife's increasingly tarnished reputation as a "bargirl." Still, Sabina's victory cannot be complete or sure. The "other" woman, valuable for bearing a child, continues to be welcomed by her in-laws and stays in the village, making a future relationship with Sabina's husband possible if not highly probable. The next section discusses the use of social aggression and the ways in which it can be much more effective in banishing rivals.

Social Aggression: Joyce and the In-Laws

A powerful example of the importance of the familial support of in-laws in defending a marriage against polygamy is demonstrated in Joyce Mhango's story. We met Joyce Mhango in the late afternoon at the end of our interviews that day. We waited for the crowd gathered for a meeting behind her house to disperse to settle on the mat with her. Mrs. Mhango is an elder and for the purposes of the village meeting had donned a bright head scarf. She coughed intermittingly but welcomed us nonetheless. In a voice weak from the coughing and tired from a long village meeting, she began to tell a story of strength.

It happened in the 1970s that her husband brought another woman to the compound and said he wanted to marry her. In this case, getting a girlfriend was not a step toward polygamy but rather a step toward dissolving his first marriage. Joyce's husband told her she should go home. Joyce returned to her natal village but was told by her family that it was not she who should leave the village but the new wife. The go-between, who acted as a kind of marriage broker and counselor, tried to settle the dispute. Joyce discovered that her brother-in-law also supported the idea that she stay in the village and that the new wife go home. However, he said, if the new wife did stay, Joyce should also stay and remarry in the same village. It seemed she had become a valued member of that family. Even her parents-in-law said that Joyce should stay. It was, in fact, only the husband who was insistent that Joyce leave. This was not enough for him to get his way.

When the case finally went to court, the husband tried to press his divorce suit, yet none of his relatives took his side. His own son, upon hearing about the divorce, testified on behalf of Joyce, his stepmother. He said, if my father does not keep Joyce and insists on taking a new wife then Joyce can come and live with me. His father could just stay with the new wife. The new wife objected to this arrangement because she had thought she would be alone in the marriage. She left. "So when the compound was in my favor, that's when she was going back." Then the husband withdrew the request for divorce. Before they began to testify at court, they said, "Nyamhango, the court does not end marriages but rather corrects marriages."

The contrast between Mrs. Mhango's case and Sabina's is striking. When Sabina sought to divest herself of her rival, she was thwarted by uncooperative in-laws who preferred the second wife to the first. They even went so far as to send Sabina back to her home. Her husband had to go against the wishes of his relatives to bring back his first wife. In Mrs. Mhango's case it was her husband who was eager to replace his current wife with a new wife. In such cases we might be tempted to think the desires of the husband would be paramount, but the overwhelming support of Joyce by his relatives secured Mrs. Mhango's place in the village. The force of their social will overcame a husband's desire to replace one wife with another. It becomes obvious that the social aggression of a collective is more effective than physical aggression in itself.

Not all acts of social pressure are as dramatically collective as Mrs. Mhango's example. Wezzie Nyasulu, one of our younger respondents, told us about a woman who went to her rival and told her that it would be a bad idea to marry her husband because of the financial struggles that already existed in his first marriage (Pauline Nyirongo, March 7, 2006). One woman, who was pregnant, went to reason with her husband's girlfriend. She was afraid her rival might have AIDS because of things she'd heard about the woman's first husband. The rival abandoned the woman's husband and married elsewhere (Masozi Nyirenda, February 20, 2006).

We heard another story about two cowives who were annoyed that their husband was bringing a third wife into the marriage. The third wife was a widow, and the two women assumed that the woman was infected with AIDS. In an expression of extreme disapproval, the mother-in-law of these women refused to eat the *nsima* of the new wife, a sign of rejection and refusal to incorporate the third wife (Grace Mwandira, January 25, 2006). Presumably such disapproval could make the woman's life so uncomfortable that she would change her mind about remaining in the marriage.

The tactic of trying to make a rival run away is not new. Lucy Mair, drawing on materials collected throughout sub-Saharan Africa in the 1940s, wrote that "there was plenty of room for jealousy between wives, expressed in an insistence on a strictly equal distribution of the husband's favors, in meanness toward the children of cowives when distributing food, sometimes in making life impossible for a new wife so that she was driven to run away to her own home" (Mair, 1953: 18). Still, individualized acts of social pressure seem less likely to yield the kind of results enjoyed by Mrs. Mhango. Mrs. Mhango's success in excluding her rival was built upon the community consensus in her favor. The era of AIDS creates a new basis for consensus as people reassess the viability of traditions such as widow inheritance and polygamy in the face of the HIV/AIDS epidemic, as demonstrated by the final case study of this chapter.

Ruth and the Widow

One of the most significant categories of people created by the HIV/AIDS epidemic is the "AIDS Widow." The AIDS widow is an archetypical figure expressed in various images and rumors circulating in Malawi and throughout sub-Saharan Africa. The reference to a widow in AIDS-era Malawi takes on connotations of danger and disease, vulnerability and need. The motif of the widow becomes mythic in the Barthian sense and brings to bear entire narratives in a single referent (Barthes, 1972). More than any other label of marginality (prostitute, spinster, foreigner), the AIDS widow may best exemplify Malawians' ambivalence toward ousting endangered outsiders. The next narrative demonstrates one woman's fear of having an AIDS widow join her marriage as a cowife.

It was early January in 2006 that we met Ruth who, like her neighbors, was in the midst of mounding and planting her maize and tobacco fields in preparation for the delayed summer rains. The day before we visited her close friend who had directed us to Ruth as someone worried about contracting AIDS from her husband. Rather than presume prior knowledge, we began by asking her if she knew of any cases of people who feared infection by a husband, and she said,

> "I am worried because when the husband started misbehaving he was sleeping with a widow so maybe during that time he took it [AIDS]...
>
> The brother of my husband is not far. The older brother of my husband was suffering from AIDS. They told us at the hospital. He suffered for three years. At that time when he was suffering he stopped sleeping with the younger wife. He would only sleep with the older wife then. Then you could see that that the elder wife got shingles. But after his death she got better and then relatives said [to my husband] you should marry her, she was not sick with AIDS, just bewitched because they were rich. Just inherit her, they were telling him. But he had been told that the brother was suffering from AIDS. Then the family was saying that my husband should marry the younger wife saying that she won't have AIDS because the husband was not sleeping with her in the end. The husband was deceived and he started going out with the younger one. That's when I started noticing a difference [in his behavior]. He started going out at eleven and people were telling me about this... When I heard people saying this he refused when I asked about it. There was a day he said "I am going to drink a bit." I became suspicious and could not sleep. So I went to see where people were drinking and saw they had left so I just went to the house of that widow. Just as I reached there I saw his leg coming from the window... He was afraid to go through the front door because there were some girls sleeping in the sitting room and he would be seen so he tried to go through the window. When I saw the leg I just caught it in my hands from the window. I said, I asked you if you had been sleeping with the widow and you said no!! But still he refused saying that I was drunk so I didn't know where I was. Besides he said, I used a condom."
>
> "Did you forgive him?" we asked.
>
> "No, I didn't forgive him. I called the relatives. The relatives, in-laws, brothers and my eldest sister and they discussed. The woman was chased away from the compound and went home."
>
> "How did that meeting go?"
>
> "After the discussion the most elder brother of my husband chased the woman saying that you are a killer. They criticized her saying that we know what our brother was suffering from. Are you trying to kill many? To finish the whole compound? The family encouraged us to go to the hospital but we have never been for a blood test because the husband refuses to go... the wife who was chased away died when

giving birth to a baby. I am afraid that maybe my husband got the disease from that woman." (Ruth Chirwa, January 2006).

Ruth's story, unlike the others, does not include a confrontation of her potential cowife. This is not to say that Ruth did not have an encounter with the "other woman" her but that this particular narrative is not about such an encounter. Instead we hear a humor-infused tale of Ruth following her husband to an assignation. We hear the story of a powerful woman taking hold of her husband by the leg as he skulks around fearfully. We see a woman who takes the dispute to her relatives and to her in-laws for mediation the result of which is the expulsion of the widow from the village. This story is about aggression against another woman but it is not about physical aggression. Instead it is about Ruth's relative power in the village among her in-laws, and it is also about the power of the AIDS Widow archetype in contemporary Malawi.

When Malawians think about widows in the time of AIDS, they think about the practice of widow inheritance. Widow inheritance is the practice of a man marrying the widow of his deceased relative. The custom is meant to afford social protection and financial support to a widow. According to some social scientists and public health officials, however, cultural practices such as widow inheritance are driving the spread of AIDS in sub-Saharan Africa. The narrative they tell is that many widows today may be so because their husbands died of AIDS. Lay people in Malawi also harbor suspicion that some widows may be infected and that by remarriage they risk further spreading HIV (Luginaah et al., 2005; Ntozi, 1997; Malungo, 2001; Luke, 2002a; 2002b; Rosenthal, 2006). In a context like Rumphi, where polygyny is common,[4] a man already married may "inherit" the wife of his relative. If this widow has HIV then the husband may potentially spread the disease to his other wives. Fear about widows is most extreme in common rumors of people who deliberately infect others so that many will follow them to the grave.

On the other hand, widows are viewed as highly vulnerable. Widow inheritance is associated with property grabbing, ritual cleansing through sexual intercourse, poverty, and dangerous social/spiritual liminality. In patrilineal communities of Northern Malawi, when a man dies his relatives can come and take the property from his widow, claiming it belongs to the family. This can leave a woman with significant financial difficulties in supporting herself and her children.

In some communities in Malawi, widow inheritance involves ritual cleansing whereby a designated member of the community must sleep with the widow to break her bond with the spirit of the dead husband. The widow as category inhabits an in-between space of the victim-villain in Malawian communities. The so-called AIDS widows are simultaneously viewed as threats to the health of the community and vulnerable members for whom the community is responsible.

All these associations and narratives are not only part of a Western discourse on African practices, but they are very much a part of Malawian AIDS education campaigning by the national government and NGOs. These stories of the deadly and victimized widow are heard on the radio, advocated by "sensitized"[5] village headmen, and preached from pulpits in sermons on charity. One informant who was monitoring media messages reported an item from the radio about a workshop where traditional leaders were being taught about the danger of certain "cultural practices":

> The workshop discussed the dangers of some cultural practices, which are fueling the spread of the virus. The traditional practices, said the chiefs of cleaning widows through sexual union and wife inheritance have no place in our area, we have declared.
>
> The traditional leaders agreed that the practice have no place in their traditions and now consider them primitive. The traditions have been banned in order to reduce the transmission of HIV among the people in the area. (Kennedy Mhango, research journal, 2006)

Not only are general narratives about inherited widows well known, but throughout Ruth's compound and the adjacent compound, several women repeated Ruth's story. One woman in Ruth's village said that the sister of the widow came to the village and warned people to "take care." The respondent went on to say that the widow had been admonished. Some people asked her to end the relationship, but according to the respondent the woman replied, "What do you think I should do and yet I don't have a husband myself?" (Masozi Nyirenda, February 2006). What is important to note here is that the respondent recognized the widow's problematic predicament. Her repetition of the widow's words might be interpreted as an expression of sympathy. The widow is not merely a dangerous "type" she is a woman who has experienced a tremendous loss of status, economic support, and security.

Discussion

In some societies gossip can be a means of storing and retrieving information from a community (Roberts, 1964: 441). The gossip known throughout the village regarding the widow's late husband became evidence against her when the case came before the elders. The collective knowledge formed in gossip was retrieved as damning evidence. Ruth was able to oust the woman from the village by deploying the powerful symbol of the widow among a community that would have immediately recognized the dangerous salience of her allusion. It is the potency of well-known AIDS stories of diseased and/or deliberately infecting widows that inhabits the widow as symbol. By deploying and invoking certain narratives, some women attempt to transform their marriages and keep their health intact.

Yet these narratives are not "just stories" in the pejorative vernacular sense of the term, these stories are rooted in experiences as evidenced by first-person narratives backed up by third-person accounts. The conventionality of fight stories and their widespread popularity should not lead us into the common fallacy of "dismiss[ing] all of the teller's claims, in advance, without the need for evidence" or negating the importance of knowing whether a real event has been reported (Hufford, 1995: 31). Fight narratives are about real social struggles. These narratives express realities and have consequences and meanings that are irreducible to words.

An outbreak of aggression between female rivals marks not only a transition of a private conflict into the public, but the fight itself can act as a declaration that a public enemy has been identified. However, a sneak attack (recall the case of Mrs. Chirwa versus Eunice, the spinster) may mark the assailed woman as victim in need of community support and Mrs. Chirwa as the underhanded aggressor. Such an outcome may in part result from the reasoning that people do evil in secret, in the darkness. Thus, women's strategies of exclusion utilize techniques of illumination, throwing light onto affairs hidden in corners. Wives using aggression make their problem a problem of the larger community. They try to create consensus around who belongs and who does not through word and deed.

What is the role of the government in the face of violence in communities? In 1994, with funding from the United Kingdom, Malawi created a special division of police called Victim Support Unit (VSU) devoted to dealing specifically with gender-based violence by providing counseling, first aid, private interviews, and referrals. The units deal mostly with cases relating to rape, defilement (child molestation), divorce, wife battery, property grabbing, and other domestic disputes including the types of domestic conflagrations this chapter highlights. The authors of a study entitled *Nkhanza*, compiled VSU records from 2000–2003 for the districts of Dedza, Mulanje, and Rumphi. *Nkhanza* is a Chichewa term encompassing multiple types of cruelty or abuse (emotional, physical, financial, sexual, etc.) including gender-based violence (Saur et al., 2000: 79). The authors found that the main interventions made by the VSUs were in the form of counseling and advice. They also found that the cases received by the VSU were not tracked much beyond referrals. However, officers offered their anecdotal observations that most women drop criminal cases due to pressure from family and friends. Some women indicated to police that going to the VSU is a move to show abusers that they are serious about wanting the abuse to stop but they ultimately have no intention of having the assailant jailed (Saur et al., 2000: 73). In the disputes recounted in this chapter, the police are rarely mentioned. Conflicts are generally dealt with by village heads, traditional authorities/chiefs, or in the immediate family without recourse to police.

In light of recent xenophobic violence in Southern Africa, it may seem dangerous and irresponsible to talk about aggression as a "strategy of exclusion" in neutral academic tones. That violence can be laughable seems revolting. On a different scale, the violence of vigilante mobs in shantytowns of South Africa could be viewed in a similar light though on a different scale of violence. Barry Bearak, a journalist writing about the killing of a Zimbabwean man by South Africans, registered the dismay of the victim's brother who wondered how people could participate in a mob killing with a sense of gaiety and celebration ("Death by a Thousand Blows," *The New York Times Magazine*, June 5, 2011). Yet somehow the act of violence itself is paradoxically an admission of the perpetrators' own vulnerability or weakness.

Women's efforts to exclude rivals can be made difficult if the "other woman" is a highly valued member of the community. The difficulty of excluding a rival is therefore contingent upon the relative social integration of the rivals and the extent to which stigmatizing labels (prostitute, AIDS widow, etc.) adhere to their subject. Complicating the matter, the struggle we witness is not necessarily between a very powerful woman and a very weak woman but between two relative equals. According to Douglas, "The histories of the definition of a disease remind us that the community also constitutes itself in a struggle for power among its members"(1991: 734). Perhaps this is why stories so amusing are at the same time so sorrowful. Laughter is part of the triumph women experiences in confronting a rival. Indeed, laughter, more specifically shared laughter, may be the only victory a woman ultimately enjoys over her rival.

CHAPTER 4

"NOBODY FEARS AIDS, *MPHUTSI* IS MORE FIRE": DISEASE RUMORS IN THE AGE OF AIDS TREATMENT

During the dry, dusty winter of 2008, a rumor caught fire in Malawi but quickly burned out. It was said that in the Southern district of Zomba, a new sexually transmitted disease was spreading. This disease, called *mphutsi*, meaning maggots, reportedly infected the genitals of its victims. Those with the disease would die rapidly—within a week or month—if they were not treated with the liver of a cow. Fear of the disease spread beyond the immediate environs of Zomba, the area believed to be at the epicenter of mphutsi infection. According to rumor, a group of men in the centrally located capital city, Lilongwe, had begun publically shouting at and tearing the clothes off prostitutes there, accusing them of spreading the disease.

Meanwhile, in the Northern district of Rumphi, a group of young Malawians arrived from various districts across the country to conduct interviews for a survey project. Some talked about mphutsi as they gathered for work. Among these survey interviewers was one of my informants, Hastings Mkandawire. He and his wife rented space to some of the people brought to work on the survey but later found out that the "wife" of one of the men they housed was not a wife but a prostitute. Hastings described a conversation that took place among himself, his wife and Charity (who he called "the hired girlfriend" of the survey worker). Hastings' wife was concerned with the women who had traveled from other regions to work on the project. She worried that Hastings might become entangled with some of those girls. Charity's discussion of a new disease did little to calm her fears. Charity explained what she had heard on the radio and why people greatly feared the spread of this particular disease:

> "AIDS is now the story of the past, nobody this time fear[s] AIDS, Mphutsi is more fire!" Charity commented. "The advantage with AIDS is that it takes a longer time before somebody kisses the ground, unlike this newly discovered disease," continued Charity who seemed to be worried very much with the disease." (Hastings Mkandawire research journal, July 2008)

The disease was believed to be inevitably fatal and incurable. Some said infected women die within a month and men within a week. Charity explained to a puzzled Hastings that women could more easily treat the disease and thus survive longer because they could place the cow's liver used for treatment inside the affected area. When Hastings chatted with a group of male research interviewers the next day, they were also talking about mphutsi. Hastings wrote that talk of the disease was "the food of everybody that day." One of the men, named Bright explained what he heard from a friend:

> "My friend phoned me yesterday, he was telling me about the same disease. He told me that at first the Malawi government through its Ministry of Health was against [acknowledging] the spread of the disease, but now it has agreed about the presence of the disease." (Hastings Mkandawire research journal, July 2008)

The same young man went on to explain that after he heard the stories about mphutsi from his friend he collected his salary but decided not to go spend it at the bottle store (bar) where he was likely to run into bargirls, that is, prostitutes. "... [M]en have to run away from bargirls, they want to protect their lives." He explained that in town there is a problem of men shouting at bargirls saying "We know you bar girls and prostitutes, you have got worms, we don't want you, you can kill us." Mphutsi, he explained, has been bad for the business of prostitution.

Around the same time Malawi's Ministry of Health published a press release in the weekend edition of *The Nation* (a nationally circulating newspaper). In their statement written to clarify facts about "a rumour of a strange disease," they began by explaining the characteristics of the sexually transmitted infection (STI):

> According to the rumour, people infected with the disease, especially women were attacked by maggots. It was further alleged that people infected with the disease were dying quickly, particularly men. (*Weekend Nation*. Ministry of Health Press Release, June 28/29)

The press release went on to assure the public that the health workers had not found any evidence of the disease in "alleged patients" and that the disease did not exist. "The Ministry of Health would, therefore, like to inform the general public that this is just a rumour and should not be a cause for anxiety" (*Weekend Nation*. Ministry of Health Press Release, June 28/29).

When I left Malawi in the July 2008 mphutsi rumors were circulating actively, but when I returned in 2010 fear of mphutsi had disappeared and new concerns were occupying the airwaves. In fact, when I spoke to other people who conducted research in Malawi between 2008 and 2010 mphutsi did not register as a concern at all. The people I interviewed in Zomba about the disease in 2010 said stories of mphutsi had circulated no more than a month or two. No general outbreak had been reported and in 2008 the Ministry of Health had publicized statements questioning the existence of the disease. One might, therefore be justified in concluding that this rumor was a mere flash in the pan, a short-lived panic unworthy of further scrutiny and certainly unworthy of scholarly attention. Yet, to relegate mphutsi rumors to unscrutinized obscurity is to miss an opportunity to glimpse the confused and searching anxieties of Malawians at a moment in history fraught with both promise and backward looking anxiety. While the disease may have not been real, the concern it aroused was. I argue that examining mphutsi rumors to understand the nature of the fear it created can grant researchers a better understanding of attitudes and beliefs about AIDS three decades into the epidemic. Furthermore, the descriptions of mphutsi's course of disease morbidity, treatment, and mortality were laid out in strikingly gendered terms. Mphutsi rumors gives voice to a persistent gendered discourse of suspicion and blame.

Concepts surrounding the origin, transmission, symptoms, and fatality of sexually transmitted diseases are bound to notions about gender roles and morality in Malawian understandings of disease. Malawians have been living with the knowledge and experience of AIDS for three decades at this point: three decades of evolving public health messages, three decades of trying to avoid infection, three decades of watching the disease take family and friends, three decades of seeking information and treatment, and three decades of providing care. As messages, coping strategies, and treatment options have evolved over time so has the experience of AIDS.

The mphutsi rumor first came to my attention while I was conducting research on a different topic in Northern Malawi in 2008. I made note of it but did not pursue field research relating to mphutsi until 2010 when I found myself in Zomba longer than I anticipated. The source material for this chapter includes my interviews with 20 individuals in a village near the city of Zomba in of 2010. I also draw from newspaper articles published in 2008, and descriptions of conversations about mphutsi written up in 2008 by two Malawian rumor journalers. My research assistant and I began our interviews in Zomba's busy market, asking simply whether people had heard of the disease and what they had heard. We were told that the person found with the disease was a prostitute who lived in a nearby village adjacent to the market. Upon being granted permission by the village head to conduct interviews, we talked to people in that particular village including several sex workers associated with the establishment where the alleged mphutsi victim was said to have worked. A third of the people we interviewed were male and the rest were female. Though they ranged in age from 20 to 50 years of age, most of the individuals we spoke to were in their 20s and 30s. The respondents were of various ethnicities (Lomwe, Chewa, Nyanja, Yao, and Tumbuka) and various professions. We interviewed salon owners, farmers, soldiers, students, pastors, merchants, commercial sex workers, and beer brewers. We found our informants as a sample of convenience, at the market or at their homes.

Assessing Beliefs in Rumors

Most informants were able to tell us something they had heard about mphutsi though some were doubtful about whether the rumors were true. So how can we assess people's attitudes toward mphutsi? If people did not unequivocally believe that mphutsi was real, why does it matter? According to Charles Rosenberg, epidemics call forth articulations of societal values as people struggle to understand their circumstances and find solutions (1987 [1962]:4). While some rumor scholars, such as sociologist Tamotsu Shibutani, suggest that rumors arise from events, Jean-Noel Kapferer suggests a different relationship of rumors to events. According to Kapferer, the rumor process is not fundamentally a representation of events that happened (Shibutani, 1966; Kapferer, 1990). Rather by engaging in the rumor process people "seek out the truth" through an assemblage of "raw, confused facts" and lay theorizing. Rumors may be thought of as collective inventions that spread because they are plausible, exciting/entertaining, and represent a shared concern or fear. One source of entertainment or fascination people experience with rumor derives from the possibility that the fantastic and shocking propositions of a story may actually represent reality. According to Luise White, what makes a rumor or legend powerful is that people believe it (White, 2000: 57). The questions we must ask, therefore, are what makes the mphutsi story shocking and what makes mphutsi stories believable? It is on the aspects that make the story seem plausible that we cast our attention.

The plausibility of a rumor is related to prior knowledge and experience of the community in which the information is circulating. Plausibility is a function of cultural context—the imagery, epistemology, and expectation of a given community. For the mphutsi rumor, the experience and knowledge of various STIs form the general epistemological groundwork for incorporating tales of a new disease. More specifically, the entrenchment and comprehensive impact of AIDS make it the central point of reference for new STIs; this chapter draws on the Malawian knowledge and experience of AIDS as a primary lens through which to interpret plausibility of mphutsi.

In addition to establishing the cultural context of rumor plausibility, rumors can be a gauge for current concerns, fears, and attitudes. They provide a "snapshot" of tangled and raw conjecture that have not been fully crystallized but nonetheless index deep cultural values and symbols. They are knowledge in the making, fusing the old with the new. Indeed, there already exists a disease called mphutsi in Malawi but the mphutsi of old seems to be quite a different animal from the one described in the rumors presented here. Morris describes the mphutsi fly as having small larva that burrow into the skin of humans and animals, causing inflammation until the larva are fully grown (at about 13 mm) and wiggle out (2004: 259). While similar in shape and sharing a name with the mphutsi of yore, 2008's mphutsi was sexually transmitted and dwelled only in the genitals of the victims. The imagery of the newer mphutsi is borrowed from the old, but it is given a new location and mode of transmission. So despite sharing a name, the newer mphutsi is best compared with HIV/AIDS. Juxtaposing long circulating discourse about AIDS with stories about mphutsi give clues to how HIV/AIDS has gone from being a new, acute crisis to a familiar/normalized chronic reality.

Origins and Transmission: The Resurrection of "Risk Categories"

Disease origin is often a central preoccupation of rumors about epidemics or new diseases. This is true in Malawi as it is elsewhere. Each community has their own list of usual suspects. Most of my informants said they heard that mphutsi came to Malawians because of the foreigners involved in the construction of the Zomba-Jali road. The Zomba-Jali-Phalombe Road (also known as M12) is aimed at connecting the city of Zomba to the estates of Mulanje to increase economic development in the area that the 101 km road will traverse. The road project is funded in part by the Malawi Government Roads Authority and in part by loans from OPEC (Organization of Petroleum Exporting Countries) through their BADEA (Banqua Arabe de Développement Economique en Afrique) and Kuwaiti funding. The roads not only connect Malawians in different regions, but because of the foreign investment and presence in building the roads they become and access point for foreign "invasion."

According to one young man, the disease was brought to Zomba *boma* through truck drivers who worked along the Jali road. Those truck drivers, he said, slept with prostitutes who worked near the construction site. Those prostitutes had previously slept with the Dutchmen working on the road. Presumably it was the Dutchmen who had brought the disease to Malawi. Another woman merely said that a Malawian prostitute slept with a "stranger" and others said that "azungu" (white people, plural of "mzungu") working on the road had brought the disease. One informant told us that he heard that a Chinese or Indian man working on the road had brought the disease. While another said that a man from Malawi's north was responsible for introducing mphutsi to Zomba. These groups or categories of people may represent significant "others" for those we interviewed in Zomba.

Epidemics bring to light important categorical divisions of the body politic (Douglas, 1966; Gilman, 1988; Goldstein, 2004). Gossip, rumor, and legend can function as social boundary markers by both defining the parameters of the group and also by articulating moral values of the group in which the talk is circulating. According to Max

Gluckman, gossip, which he defines as talking about other people's business, is a way people mark themselves off as a group and thereby maintain that group (Gluckman, 1963). We can extend the notion of boundary making to larger constituencies (like those who consider themselves Malawian or even African) in which rumors find their relevance. Mary Douglas describes the body as the central metaphor for the social body such that "...ideas about separating, purifying, demarcating and punishing transgressions have their main function to impose system on an inherently untidy experience" (Douglas, 1966: 3–4). During times of epidemic or even times of rumors about epidemics, the rumor process becomes a source of collective boundary making—the sort of boundary making that seeks to mark off the sick from the well, "us" from "them," insiders from outsiders. The physically sick are viewed as transgressing moral codes. The moral and the medical are therefore inextricably implicated in one another in everyday talk.

While white, Chinese, and Indian as categories may each be important individual categories for people in Zomba, perhaps the association these groups have in common in the Malawian imagination is that of "foreigners with money." That is they are non-Malawians or non-Africans whom they perceive as more wealthy than Malawians or "Africans." The very mobility of these foreigners and their presence in Malawi is evidence of wealth. The ability of people from other nations to move between countries and for other nations to fund development projects, which Malawi's government cannot fund, attests to their greater wealth. So too are the individuals involved in those development projects perceived as wealthier. Afterall, road workers have wage employment while many Malawians struggle to find such work.

In fact, the usage of particular categories (white, Indian, Chinese, Dutch, etc.) was less consistent across interviews than was the reference to the Zomba-Jali road construction project itself and to money. While some people referenced specific foreigners, more simply mentioned that it was road contractors who had brought the disease. Inherent in the notion of someone having "brought the disease" is the idea that it was brought from an "other" place. However, by not referencing a specific place or people group we get the notion that it is more important that mphutsi has been brought and is from elsewhere than where exactly it came from. It is more important that mphutsi is not of Malawi origins or due to Malawian transgressions. It is more important that mphutsi is associated with the road, mobility, foreigners, and development than it is to pin down exactly which foreign others are responsible for mphutsi.

The road as a symbol in the Central/Southern African region has potent associations. The way in which good roads compress travel time and create links and access between distant lands has both positive and negative connotations for Malawians. Desire for increased commerce, mobility, and connectivity to wider areas is offset by fears of evils that lurk on the road. Malawian discourses reveal a fear of undesirable foreign influences, the potential for foreign extraction (as exemplified in colonial practices), and the misuse of roads by Malawian witches or Satanists seeking to boost their own power and wealth by causing deadly road accidents. Besides the threat of disruptive social, cultural, and spiritual influences of foreign or modernizing elements, the road also creates a way for foreign pathogens to find a home in Malawians. The mobile populations that traverse the roads (traders, soldiers, truck drivers, etc.) or the people who serve those populations (e.g., prostitutes) have previously been under scrutiny as the "at risk" populations that brought HIV/AIDS to Malawi. Prostitutes have attracted a great deal of the blame in the public discourse surrounding AIDS:

> The identity of sex workers—that is, the ways in which they are publicly discussed and officially depicted cannot be disaggregated at this point, in other words, from pervasive understandings of the AIDS epidemic. Notions of sex workers as dangerous extends as well to the more general rubric of promiscuity, particularly as this describes women. The example above of Malawian youth's associations of risk with prostitution exemplifies the degree to which public discourses have melded social identity with infectious status. The inevitable outcome of this association is a greater blame relegated to girls and women for the transmission of HIV. (Craddock, 2000: 161)

Similarly, Malawians who were blamed for mphutsi were said to act as bridges between the foreign originators and the general population of Malawians. Prostitutes were consistently identified as possible "bridge" populations that could carry the disease from rich foreigners to the Malawian general population. The blame prostitutes received relates to popular ideas about gender and sexuality. According to one young man we interviewed the road workers were compelled by the nature of their work to fall for the temptation of prostitutes:

> If we look at social [context], those people [men constructing the road] were staying alone somewhere else and they were generating income and then they attracted these sexual workers. That is how I look at it and for sure they [commercial sex workers] were enticed by the money which were there and then you [know] how it goes (Charles Gama, Malawi, July 2, 2010)

In Malawi, there is a strongly held belief that men "cannot just stay" without having sex for a long period of time (see also Kaler (2003) and Watkins (2004: 682). As a result it is almost taken for granted that a man who spends long periods of time away from his wife/wives or girlfriend(s) will have sexual partners elsewhere. This irresistible force of man's nature removes some of the sting of blame from men who are unfaithful during their travels. You cannot blame a man for being a man in the face of temptation. Indeed, in the above quote the men are not running after temptation but the relative affluence of the male road workers "attracted these sexual workers." It is the women who sexually tempt men that are be blamed. With respect to the AIDS epidemic, anthropologists working in the Zomba region have pointed out disproportionate blame that fell upon women when AIDS prevalence rates began to skyrocket (Peters, Kambewa, and Walker, 2010). The mphutsi rumor continues or revives that tradition. Indeed, two young men we interviewed, Bester Musa and Happy Msowoya, said that mphutsi was a punishment to prostitutes.

Bester: That mphutsi was in Zomba it was true (laughs). To me I believe it was a punishment to these prostitutes

Anika: Okey, it was to punish the prostitute then?

Bester: Yes, we say so because the woman they suspected was like a prostitute you know. And at the road contraction [construction] there are always prostitutes and at the end of the day because there is money.

Msowoya: Yeah, people come back [from working road construction] with a lot of money and not people from the village there. And I feel it is just a punishment to these prostitutes.

Anika: Does it mean that it [mphutsi] was not spreading to those people [from the village] then? But specifically to the people who were doing prostitution then?

Bester: No. I think this disease was not spread in the entire village, no. There were just few individuals, two or three people. But it was this man who was spreading this disease. That is what I heard.

Anika: Okey, so there was one man who was spreading [it]?

> *Bester*: Yeah, there was one man and I believe he was not a Malawian but he stays in Zomba just because of road construction.
>
> (Happy Msowoya and Bester Musa, July 2, 2010)

Bester draws clear boundaries between the innocent population of the village and the prostitutes and foreign road constructors who infect them. The excerpt above mentions prostitutes and their culpability for spreading the disease but interprets their infection further as a punishment for tempting men and taking their money. Indeed, Bester's statements express the sense that the disease is targeted toward these women somehow. No one else from the village from which the prostitutes come was infected. One young woman we interviewed, Beatrice Ntaja, said, "because she [the person infected with mphusti] was a prostitute she got the disease through having multiple partners...[There was] no specific person she got the disease from [but rather from] the thing that she does. She is a prostitute. She sleeps with many people" (Beatrice Ntaja, July 2, 2010). The woman's activities had generated the maggots. She slept with too many people. There is a similar belief about AIDS; people feel that those who get AIDS are those who have too much sex with too many partners (Peters, Kambewa, and Walker, 2008: 662).

AIDS also had similar reputation as a population-specific disease that moved relatively quickly from predominance in "at risk" bridge groups like soldiers, truckers, and prostitutes into the general population. Although the first diagnosis of the disease in Malawi was made in 1985, by 1994 there were 36,236 reported cases (Walden et al., 1999). Yet by the early 2000s it was becoming clear that HIV/AIDS was inflicting many more than just those in occupations labeled risky or mobile. The newspaper *Malawi Nation* published an article highlighting the risk to a broad swath of the population:

> Aids has graduated from a shocking phenomenon to a grim fact of life. Once restricted to a few countries and *specific populations* [my emphasis added], today AIDS and the HIV which causes Aids effects men, women and children of all ages everywhere. (*Malawi News*, Rotary to aid Aids victims, November 27, 2001)

As the HIV/AIDS prevalence rate rose to a height of 14% of the population for those between 15–49 by 2004, it became increasingly impossible to separate the sick from the well. If early in the epidemic AIDS seemed a disease of foreign homosexuals, mobile segments of the local population (such as soldiers, truckers, and traders), and commercial sex workers, in the new millennium, it is all too clear that everyone in Malawi is either "affected or infected" by HIV/AIDS.[1]

By contrast, there is a comforting simplicity to this configuration of mphutsi in which those designated as "guilty" suffer alone. Unlike AIDS, which is commonly described by Malawians as a disease that has come to kill everyone, mphutsi punishes a few, only those worthy of being punished. Indeed, most people said they only heard of between one and three individuals being infected with mphutsi. This is not the experience Malawians have known with HIV/AIDS. Yet, the experience of AIDS transforming from a disease of the few blameworthy "at risk" to a disease of the general population inhabits the fear evident in mphutsi rumors. In this context, it is very plausible fear for people to believe that mphutsi (if it had proved to be real) could move out of the at risk population to anyone.

Whereas the specter of AIDS animated fear of mphutsi, mphutsi expresses a muted or subdued fear of AIDS. As quoted at the beginning of this chapter: "[N]obody this time fear[s] Aids, mphutsi is more fire!" The rumors themselves suggest several explanations for this muted fear of AIDS including the "normalizing" of AIDS in everyday life over time and the increased availability of ARVs in Malawi resulting in lengthened progression from infection to death. In addition, the veiled visibility of AIDS as compared to mphutsi was stressed in these rumors with great ambivalence. These themes are explored in the following sections.

AIDS as the New Normal

As it has become increasingly impossible and (undesirable) for Malawians to "separate, demarcate, and punish transgressors" (Douglas, 1966: 3–4), AIDS has settled into the fabric of everyday life. Contrary to public health campaigns and predictions, those who have AIDS in Malawi generally have not been ostracized, stigmatized, or rejected from their communities. Public health officials, NGOs, and the media in Malawi frequently allude to an atmosphere of "denial" and claim that people living with AIDS are stigmatized by their communities. Yet, extensive qualitative research has shown that Malawians neither reject the reality of AIDS nor jettison those infected from their communities,[2] instead people have been "trying to control the abnormal circumstances of the rising toll of

HIV-related illness and death, making huge efforts to channel them into the normal and normative ways of their society" (Peters et al., 2008: 662).

Another sign of AIDS normalization is found in the domestication or "vernacularization" of HIV/AIDS prevention strategies. Susan Watkins' research describes the Malawian development of HIV/AIDS avoidance strategies that are modifications or variations on public health recommendations (2004). Public health messages telling people to "abstain, be faithful, and use condoms" are modified in a society in which sexual intercourse is seen as healthy and necessary activity. Instead of strictly following the advice of public health officials, men and women reduce their number of partners and take care in selecting partners by relying upon the reputation of their potential lovers and an assessment of their physical appearance (2004). Others leave marriages with partners who they believe are putting them in danger (Reniers, 2003). Men and women continue to care for their sick and incorporate orphans into their extended-family households (Chimwaza and Watkins, 2004). People are trying to carry on in as "normal" a fashion as possible with an epidemic in their midst that does not seem to be going anywhere soon.

The adjustment to and "normalization" of AIDS in Malawi over time has made it possible to conceive of mphutsi, a disease that sets "at risk" people apart, as simultaneously comforting and terrifying. That, according to rumor, only the two or three blameworthy and marginal community members get sick, is perhaps a welcome change from a disease that has "come for all people" according to local discourse. But because the descriptions of mphutsi's origins and mode of transmission were similar to those of HIV, it is terrifying. Sexually transmitted, brought by foreigners, transmitted to Malawian prostitutes and mobile workers, and inevitably deadly. The echoes of early AIDS discourse are clear and the fear of a potential for wider generalized epidemic can be assumed even when unspoken. The parallels are too striking to think otherwise. The potential for a general outbreak was part of the brief terror stirred by mphutsi. Yet to understand further the fear stirred by mphutsi, it is necessary to examine discussions about the symptoms and timeline from infection to death. While mphutsi is comforting in the simplicity of categories, it is terrifying in the frightful symptoms through which it accomplishes its boundary making. The idea of visible worms spewing out of the genitals is a shocking image of death by consumption made visible that is explored further in the next section. The next section deals specifically with descriptions of mphutsi symptoms.

Mphutsi: An Obvious Sign of Death in the Body

In this section, I focus on two symptoms of mphutsi that drew comparison to AIDS and were manifested in gendered ways: the visibility of the disease on the body and the timeline from disease presentation to death. Compared to AIDS, mphutsi was described as a disease that made itself known as a sexually transmitted disease through obvious and evocative symptoms: maggots issuing directly from the genitals. The hiddenness of the HI virus before one develops full-blown AIDS causes great concern, speculation, and gossip, yet, the alternative of radical visibility of mphutsi symptoms and rapid progression to death seemed even more terrifying.

The notion of the invisibility of mphutsi is alluded to when people discuss stories about disease "carriers," people who are infected with a disease and can transmit it to others but do not succumb to sickness or death themselves. The stories of carriers had a strikingly gendered character such that men especially were said to "carry" the disease invisibly and infect women who would then suffer visible symptoms. A young man, Fred Byson, a second-year student at the Malawi College of Health Sciences in Zomba, said that he heard that a woman from the village of Chikanda had the "so-called disease" (his designation) and that she got the disease from a man who was infected but showed no signs of illness. Indeed, said Byson, the disease was similar to the virus that causes cervical cancer in women but no illness in men (Fred Byson, June 30, 2010). Other informants reported a modified version of the "carrier" theory saying that mphutsi was a disease from which women predominantly suffered. One woman explicitly said that it was "a disease for women" (Ruth Mpoya, July 1, 2010). One man claimed that women were more affected than men because it was women who would develop symptoms (Daniel Chisale, July 2, 2010). Bula Matola, a young woman who worked as a commercial sex worker at the bar where an mphutsi victim was rumored to work, said it was women only were infected.

> *Bula*: Men were just like carriers and deposit to a woman. A woman could be known [to have the disease].

Anika: A man couldn't die from this?
Bula: A man could just be a carrier or else he could not be affected as a woman could be affected. (Bula Matola, July, 2010)

Despite the predominance of the men carrier/women sufferer configuration, beliefs about who suffered from the disease were not uniform. Mina Chitende, who is a vendor at the market, said that men and women are infected at equal rates but only women suffer from the symptoms of the disease (Mina Chitende, June 30, 2010).

People who believe that men are carriers and not sufferers of mphutsi touch upon the problem of hidden disease, a problem familiar to people from their experience with AIDS and other sexually transmitted diseases known in the region. Much talk about AIDS in Malawi has centered around trying to discern which people in the community are infected with AIDS based on piecing together their sexual histories and illness histories through hearsay and observation. The tentative conclusions people reach in this piecing together becomes the basis of decisions in acquiring sexual partners and spouses (Watkins, 2004). The fear of a disease carrier whose internal illness is masked by a relatively healthy appearance has been a major source of HIV/AIDS gossip- and rumor-mongering. The quote below from the Malawi Diffusion and Ideational change Project (also known as "Let's Chat") journal project exemplifies a common way of talking about people believed to have HIV/AIDS. A group of men at a bar discuss the HIV status of a woman's whose beauty is believed to mask a deadly secret:

> "Do you see that woman who is dancing there?" [says one man]. And his friend saw her attentively and that man continued, "That woman is from Tswingwe, she started prostitution long ago and some of her friends [other prostitutes] she was playing with while doing this, they are all no more but she is still strong up to now." Then his friend said, "But if you can meet her on the way for the first time without knowing her properly you can't know that she is poison, you can just think that you have found an enjoyable woman." Then the first man said, Komani! Having sex with that woman is just a careless manner and it is better to dip your member in acid because you can have the developed sores cured [rather] than going for that woman. And his friend said, "But looking at her health, you can't know about all that." And the first man said, "Some people are just carriers so that they do catch this AIDS but not suffer from it themselves but

> those who do go for them, they do catch the disease and I think that this woman can be of that kind. (Diston Geladi MDICP research journaler, September 10, 2003)

The external signs of the woman's health are described as deceptive. In reality her body is a site of danger and death to others. Men were also described as being carriers of HIV. One journaler described a conversation that took place among several men at a beer hall. The men observed the activities of a man who was thought to be an AIDS carrier and nicknamed "The Machine" or "The Grinding Machine." The Machine was a man who was said to be able to sleep with (grind) many women in succession and destroy (grind) them by way of infecting them with HIV without himself becoming ill. Unlike the prostitute "carrier" described in the previous excerpt, The Machine does not enjoy a natural immunity to HIV but instead is privileged by access to anti-retroviral medicine. ARVs are a twist on the gossip and warnings about disease carriers in communities. One of the men at the bar opined, "He looks strong and healthy because he has money, the ARVs are helping him otherwise he would have been dead by now, explained George." ARVs create the illusion of health and make it difficult for observers to read the signs of illness. This means that without a recitation of the subject's sexual reputation people could be deceived by visual cues about the health of The Machine (Magwira, MDICP research journaler, July 6, 2005).

As illustrated above, the Malawian conception of disease "carrier" is flexible. In some cases, people talk about disease carriers as if they are immune while others refer to disease carriers as those who are infected but whose illness is delayed either naturally by the slow course of the disease or artificially through the use of medical interventions. For those who wish to identify people living with HIV/AIDS, the problem of a lack of visual cue to illness is also created by the lag time between infection and visibly observable illness episodes. Mphutsi, however, resolves this dilemma. Mphutsi illness is said to come swiftly on the heels of transmission. One person we interviewed remarked, "The person (woman) slept with another man and the next morning the man noticed-really!-that he was releasing mphutsi." (Beatrice Ntaja, July 2, 2010). Added to this rapid development of disease in the body is both the radical visibility of the disease and the subsequent rapid descent into death.

The shocking visibility of mphutsi was a major point of concern among those we interviewed. When we asked one woman whether AIDS or mphutsi was scarier she said that mphutsi was because "[w]hen you sit down the disease shows but with AIDS it does not show. [You] can be totally embarrassed." The maggots were not only a visible sign of disease and the moral sickness but also certain sign that death resided in the bodies of the infected.

> *Charles*: People were just saying oh I need to change my behavior because of the issue. That's what many people were saying because just imagine seeing that mphutsi coming out of the body—that was something very scary! You don't even imagine yourself being alive, you will think that you are dead or something. [Daniel Chisala, another respondent, laughs] Do you know what I mean by that? So it made people change their behaviors. (Charles Gama, July 2, 2010)

Mphutsi was described as indisputable proof of moral culpability. In this case, the larva seems not as the kind that burrow into the living (as the mphutsi of old) but the type of maggots that feed upon decaying carrion. The decay was immediate as signaled by automatic production of maggots that eat the flesh of the dead.

There are similarities to be found with AIDS discourse in that people have described HIV/AIDS as death abiding stubbornly in bodies. It is there lurking even when not visible. During my research in Malawi between 2004 and 2008, there were times when I heard people with AIDS described as the "walking dead" and those who are "dead but alive." And perhaps most poignantly it has been said that "We these days move half dead." (Mkandawire research journal, August 12, 2005). The potency of AIDS in Malawian discourse resides (in part) in its entrenchment and durability in bodies combined with a long incubation period in which the presence of the disease is not apparent to onlookers. The lack of cure means that AIDS stays with you forever. This has been a frightening fact of the disease for a long time but this fear may have started to become muted recently. Since 2005 Malawi's government hospitals have drastically increased the availability of life-prolonging drugs. The next section deals with the time dimension of mphutsi rumors. More specifically I examine ways that the fears expressed over mphutsi's rapid timeline from infection to death make apparent an embrace of ARV treatment by Malawians.

"There Is Time to Die": Treatment and Time with AIDS and Mphutsi

When asked whether AIDS or mphutsi was worse one respondent replied that the feelings were mixed on the issue because with AIDS one takes time to die:

> *Simon*: People had mixed feelings on the thing. If you compare to AIDS, AIDS is something that is talked about every day and people also know that when you contract AIDS you don't die instantly. Many people cannot even know you [have AIDS]. Looking at what is happening these days you can always look healthy this and that but that situation with mphutsi [CS laughs] you cannot eat! You cannot sleep! You cannot even tell anyone of your condition. You can even have trouble moving around—they [maggots] can even fall down. That is something—no one can believe you—very shameful. I can say...people were very scared on this one [more] than AIDS. Of course, AIDS is a killer but once you have it there is time to die. (Charles Gama, July 2, 2010)

When one has "time to die" one also has time to live. By contrast, mphutsi was described as a disease that killed quickly after infection, without a lengthy incubation period. The different time frame is an important area of comparison between mphutsi and AIDS.

For AIDS patients in the global North, AIDS was transformed from an acute disease into a chronic illness around 1996 through the development of a three drug combination course generically referred to as antiretroviral therapy (ART). Those who took antiretroviral medicines (ARVs) could manage their viral load after they had entered the phase of "full blown AIDS," a phase that had previously been characterized by rapid decline, illness, and death. While the global north saw a steady decline in death rates from AIDS, those living in poorer corners of the world found themselves shut out of effective treatment by the pricing of the ARVs by pharmaceutical companies. At the same time, word of the improvements in treatment therapies spread to impoverished countries even while the drugs themselves did not. In Malawi, rumors and conspiracy theories circulated at the turn of the millennium positing a deliberate withholding of medicines by pharmaceutical corporations in collusion with rich nations. It was said that these entities sought to "control" the population of poor countries in hopes that they would no longer "beg" rich countries for money. Other rumors suggested that the medicines were only for the rich individuals and politicians they witnessed getting "fat" or flying to South Africa or Europe for treatment. People complained that there was no way a poor person could afford those drugs that were not only costly but also no cure and needed to be taken on a monthly basis (Wilson, 2008).

Before 2001, the cost of ARVs in Malawi ran between MK10,000–30,000 (about 135–415 USD) per month—far beyond the reach of most Malawians. After negotiations took place between the World Health Organization, pharmaceutical companies, and representatives of both richer and poorer countries, the cost of ARVs dropped to MK4,500 per month (about 50 USD) and then again to about MK2,500 per month (about 28 USD) making the life-prolonging drugs much cheaper but still out of reach of many Malawians. In 2003, the World Health Organization launched an ambitious program aimed at reaching three million eligible AIDS patients in poor countries with ART by the year 2005. The Government of Malawi applied as a "resource poor country" and received funding from the Global Fund to Fight AIDS, Tuberculosis, and Malaria that allowed them to supply ARVs at no cost to patients beginning in 2004 with a small number of patients and expanding to approximately 200,000 by 2009 (HIV and AIDS Monitoring and Evaluation Report, 2008–2009). Malawi and other countries that benefited from the negotiations for lowering prices on ARVs have recently begun to see the results in lower HIV transmission rates and AIDS-related deaths (UNAIDS 2011 World AIDS Day Report).

In the last seven years, regular Malawians (read: non-elite and not rich) began to experience and observe for the first time in their everyday lives the potential for AIDS to become a chronic disease as it has become in the world's richer nations. Yet even with the scale up of ARV availability in Malawi the fact remains that the drugs do not eliminate the disease from the body and that those who take them must go monthly to administering government hospitals to replenish their supplies. The government's efforts to supply free drugs have certainly reduced some of the financial onus from individual drug procurement and the related fears about the continuity of supply. Yet, the government has also had difficulties in maintaining a steady supply of drugs with reports of failures in the supply chain and shortages in hospitals. All these difficulties of cost and continuity may be reflected in mphutsi rumors. Like AIDS, one of the distinguishing features of mphutsi is that it has no cure but rather a treatment that must constantly be replenished in order to be effective. While some informants said they had not heard of a cure or treatment for mphutsi, some told us that the only way to treat the disease was to apply liver to the affected area. Below I include the remarks of several informants:

> The symptoms were larva coming down from the vagina but if people wanted to live longer they would get offals [liver] from a goat or cow so that larva would feed on those instead than on herself. If she did not put those offals she could die within a week. (Bula Matola, July 3, 2010)
>
> You needed to put a liver there or the larva would eat the person. To reduce risk they would put a liver there, when that finishes (with the liver), they would put another. (Mina Chitende, June 30, 2010)
>
> The medicine is the liver from a cow. They would insert the liver so the larva would be feeding on the *chiwindi* [liver] . . . People were complaining because of no cure and just needed to use liver . . . People were not even sure that *chiwindi* worked. (Baina Chilembe, July 1, 2010)
>
> The people at the hospital examined a woman who was said to have mphutsi but they did not find it. Only the woman who died [in Jali] had the disease. She got the disease from *mzungu* who said he would give her 30,000 MK [about 200 USD] every month for buying *chiwindi* to treat the disease . . . The *mzungu* could manage [the cost] but she died [anyway]. (Emma Willard, July 1, 2010)

According to the women quoted above, the only rumored treatment for mphutsi was liver from a cow or goat. The larvae were hungry to eat human flesh but the livers of cows or goats were an appropriate but expensive substitutes. However, many Malawians have diets that are not rich in animal proteins and whose finances disallow the purchase or slaughter of cattle on a frequent basis (UN World Food Program 2010 "Rural Malawi Comprehensive Food Security and Vulnerability Analysis").

The substitution of a woman's flesh for that of a cow's innards has other interesting connotations. First, cattle (goats and cows) are used as bridewealth by some in Malawi to secure sexual access to a woman and to her reproductive capacity. However, in the predominantly matrilineal Southern region (where these interviews were conducted) cash is used rather than cattle. Despite this, even matrilineal peoples are familiar with the practice of bridewealth involving the transfer of cattle from the family of the groom to the family of the bride.

The liver treatment for mphutsi may be said to play on this imagery. Secondly, sex is associated with "eating" in Malawi such that we may discern another type of substitution. According to the moral economy of mphutsi rumors, the hunger for money that leads women to offer themselves up to be "eaten" by strangers also leads to their total consumption by the mphutsi. The hunger for money has turned in on the women to consume them totally. The only escape now being to substitute the costly parts of a cow or goat in the place of their own bodies. Ironically, this becomes a financially ruinous and impossible undertaking as most people in Malawi cannot afford the cost of constantly replenishing livers to feed voracious mphutsi.

AIDS has also been described as a hungry disease that eats a person. In 2008, research journaler from Northern Malawi wrote about a conversation in which he, his father, and a friend gossip about the possible AIDS status of their relative, Kakoba. Mkandawire's father described the man as formerly "tall and fat" and now "tall and thin" and very likely suffering from AIDS. Hastings Mkandawire, the journaler, protested

> "So you think it is AIDS? Do you mean to say that other diseases can't eat the flesh of somebody and anybody you see thin after illness, you automatically think it is AIDS? There are other diseases as TB and Malaria which also eat the flesh of people. You can only know that somebody is suffering from HIV/AIDS after testing." (Mkandawire research journal, 2008)

AIDS, as well as other diseases "eat" the flesh of their hosts, wasting their bodies to thinness. With mphutsi the microscopic virus of AIDS is replaced with the visible larva of a fly.

Just as mphutsi and AIDS are both described as diseases that consume the body, treatments for both diseases are similarly inaccessible due to cost. The need to be rich to treat mphutsi echoes a not-so-long-ago problem Malawians had with accessing antiretroviral medicine. The high cost coupled with the necessity of replenishing the drugs on a regular basis made the idea of ARV treatment inconceivable to the average Malawian previous to the government scale up (Wilson, 2008: 72–105). Several of the Let's Chat journalists mentioned these concerns:

> One [man] said that the drugs are so expensive and are only for the rich people because they can afford to buy them every month because

> once you start taking it you have to make sure that you are taking it every month once and failing which then just know that you can't stay longer before you die of it. (Simon Bato, MDICP research journal, December, 2003)
>
> "But AIDS has no cure,' came in Nyachihana, she further added [...] "You could stop [taking ARVs] to become sick time and again but the virus won't come out of you." (Lilyan Dambo, MDICP research journal, December, 2005)

Like AIDS, mphutsi was described as having no cure. The maggots could be drawn out of the body with liver but that was not seen as a definitive cure. Instead, people have to take drugs for the rest of their lives in order to survive. "You eat, they eat" said Catherine, summarizing the comments of our informant as he spoke about the parasitic and enduring infection of mphutsi. As long as your life is extended, so is the life of the parasite.

The concern with costly food to feed a disease may also reflect concerns with the dietary recommendations for people being treated with ARVs. Research suggests that the survival rate of people on ARVs is diminished if they do not receive proper nutrition for the absorption of the medications and the reduction of side effects (UNAIDS 2008 HIV, Food Security and Nutrition; Paton 2006). The concern that ARVs should be coupled with adequate nutrition has circulated widely in Malawi's mass media and informal conversations. One old man in Rumphi had a long list of complaints about ARVs that he expressed in the presence of one of the Rumphi rumor journalers. One of his complaints was about the need for good food with drug treatment:

> And the other thing is that you will find out that we get free ARVs from the western countries. Yet people cannot take ARVs without having food. [I] Hope you all know that a lot of people are dying in Africa because they take ARVs yet they don't eat [food] which is rich in making their bodies to be strong or healthy. (Simon Nyirenda research journal, December 16, 2005)

Another journaler from Rumphi summarized a Malawi Broadcast Company (MBC) radio broadcast from January 2006, which featured comments from people living with AIDS:

> "Our bodies need food most of the time and good food, especially when we take drugs. So, we are complaining that drugs can't be

> effective if we don't eat properly most of us are poor, therefore we can't afford to buy soft foods which are required, said Arnold Zungu recently one of the people living with HIV in Mzimba.
>
> Rose Zgambo, who is one of the people living with HIV in Rumphi also concurs with Zungu, saying it is sad that many people are dying because their bodies lack strength because of shortage of food nutrients." (Kennedy Mhango research journal, January 17, 2006)

AIDS is a hungry disease that eats you. It is a disease said to make its sufferers hungry as is evidenced in a conversation from a Balaka District (Southern Malawi) journaler report in which a group of men laughed about how AIDS affected people's appetites and causes them to crave meat, especially meat fried in oil, a luxury (Simon Bato, MDICP research journal, January 4, 2003). The most effective treatment, ARVs, is also very hungry treatment that demands expensive food. So one may receive free drugs but find that they need more and better food to sustain the treatment thereby draining their resources. Mphutsi is similarly hungry as a disease, demanding an expensive treatment that must be eaten constantly. Mphutsi is the fear of insatiable AIDS and ARVs intensified, visualized, and on a compressed timeline.

Women at Work, Women "at Risk"

While AIDS gives one "time to die" mphutsi hurtles people toward their death in great haste, discriminating between men and women in doing so. At the beginning of this chapter, I presented information from Malawi's Department of Health press release in which the agency said that mphutsi was believed to infect women more often but kill men faster. Men are said to die within a week while women may take up to a month. This configuration of gendered suffering poses complications for analysis. Who is being punished here? Who is being held accountable? Are their innocent victims in these scenarios? This notable gender bias in the progression of mphutsi leads us to not only consider questions of culpability but also to look at the issue of vulnerability. In the case of mphutsi, it seems that women are said to more easily infected but men to die more quickly. If we take AIDS as the dominant reference then to what is being referred in this configuration?

A number of scholars who have chronicled the history of anti-AIDS programming in sub-Saharan Africa have shown how many programs unintentionally reified categories of guilty or vulnerable women (Booth, 2004; Hunter, 2010; Schoepf, 2001). While prostitutes have been labeled as "reservoirs" of disease, rural wives and mothers (with husbands migrating between town and country) have been described as innocent victims (Booth, 2004: 94). Women in general are portrayed as more susceptible socially, economically, and biologically. Women have been perceived as socially disempowered or vulnerable vis-a-vis husbands and elders who wield significant influence over decision-making relating to sex and child bearing. In these negotiations, women may find themselves unable to demand the use of condoms or reduce the number of children without secretly obtaining birth control. Women who cannot say "no" to sex with a possibly infected spouse find themselves at increased risk of contracting sexually transmitted diseases besides HIV, which in turn increase their susceptibility to contracting HIV. Women have less access to income and wage generating opportunities than men in Malawi. Biologically, women are more likely to contract HIV during intercourse with a man than a man is to contract HIV from a woman. The public health community both internationally and on the local level in Malawi helped to foster the image of innocent victims in the forms of babies, wives, widows, and orphans.

The tendency to perceive women "at risk" as either innocent mother-madonnas or as prostitute-whores is revisited in the mphutsi scare. However, mphutsi rumors play most directly with the prostitute image by alluding to women's biological susceptibility to HIV while simultaneously blaming women who have sex in exchange for money as potential disease spreaders. In this scenario, the women are biologically vulnerable and socially/morally culpable. Yet, what makes them susceptible (their vaginas or female reproductive organs more generally) also gives infected women a greater ability to be treated for mphutsi with liver. It is unclear whether the greater longevity of mphutsi-afflicted women compared to mphutsi-afflicted men owes primarily to ideas about gender-differentiated efficacy of treatment or whether the disease just kills women more slowly. However, if we take women's greater longevity with mphutsi as a function of treatment then this aspect of the rumor may share some echo of AIDS treatment history in Malawi. Free antiretroviral medicines (ARVs) were first available to pregnant women at antenatal clinics in 2001 (Kasenga, 2010) to prevent mother-to-child transmission during birth and later free ARVs were available to Malawi's general population in early 2004 (Libamba et al., 2007). It is the "innocents"—mothers and infants—of the AIDS epidemic that first received free access to life-prolonging ARVs. With mphutsi rumors it is the "guilty" sex workers that have the chance to prolong their lives because they are women.

Despite the persistent circulation and reification of ideas about differences between "mothers" and "whores," the reality of women's identities in sub-Saharan Africa is more complex:

> The virtual obsession with women who could be identified as prostitutes and the inability to see that such women were probably not part of clearly bounded sexual communities are the effects, in part, of the migration of the Euro-American model. Twenty years after the start of the epidemic and in the face of very high rates of the infection in nearly every community, it is still common to assume that AIDS comes from prostitutes, that "good" women will not get infected, and that if such women do become HIV positive either they were prostitutes after all or their men were engaging in risky behaviors with prostitutes. (Booth, 2004: 99)

According to this configuration, the innocent women being treated may not be perceived as ultimately innocent afterall. If mphutsi is interpreted as a punishment of a man against prostitutes (as one informant described it) then the vigilante who spreads the disease is fulfilling a role that the government has not. Over the decades of the AIDS epidemic in Malawi, rumors and gossip about deliberate HIV transmitters have arisen. In this type of rumor someone who has HIV and who is doomed to die decides that he or she does not want to die alone but wants to take as many others with them to the grave as they possibly can. The concern about deliberate HIV transmitters has lead to recurring debates about whether there should be a law against purposefully spreading HIV (WLSA 2009 Malawi CEDAW Shadow Report). Mphutsi rumors suggest that while women may be punished for tempting men, they can also use their vulnerability to their advantage in accessing treatment. The rumors also suggest that someone who is guilty of what should be a crime according to popular opinions (deliberately spreading disease) could also be doing humanity a favor.

This type of thinking helps to put in perspective the January 2012 events in the cities of Lilongwe and Blantyre wherein male vendors attacked women walking down the street for wearing trousers instead of skirts or dresses. Trousers on women are perceived by many in Malawi as sexually provocative, causing men to fall into sexual temptation. Under the Banda regime women were banned from wearing trousers. This ban was lifted in 1994 with the transition to multiparty democracy. But the issue of trousers on women continues to be contentious. During a large conference for Christian youth in March 2006 I observed a question and answer session with group leaders in which one of the teens asked them whether it was a sin for women to wear trousers. A newspaper article entitled "Tight trousers spreading AIDS" explored the debates among participants of a Central Church of Africa Presbyterian (CCAP) AIDS workshop in Karonga District.

One of the participants, Witness Munthali, a respected woman at Chilumba, said tight trousers have contributed greatly to the spread of HIV and AIDS because women deliberately wear them to seduce men. "Women deliberately wear tight trousers to tempt men. And men, weak as they are, sleep with the women thereby spreading the Aids virus." (*The Nation*, May 2006).

In the January 2012 attack, some trousered women were beaten and stripped. Apparently the AIDS scapegoat is back and she's wearing tight jeans. The events lead to a protest in Blantyre and prompted the president and vice president to give statements saying that women could wear whatever they want according to the law. One woman who participated in protests following the attacks was interviewed by the BBC and said, "Trousers and mini-skirts for most women in Malawi is a symbol for our hard-won freedom from the one-party dictatorship to the multiparty era" (*BBC News Africa*, January 20, 2012).

Because women were said to live longer than men with mphutsi, the rumors might be said to constitute a revenge fantasy of women against men. However, this aspect of the rumor better resembles the ideas of women's bodies (particularly sex worker's bodies) as repositories of disease; prostitutes spread HIV and mphutsi incidentally as part of their work. Their ability to live longer with mphutsi is a matter of anatomical "convenience" that allows better administration of mphutsi treatment. On the balance, however, it is women who proved most vulnerable in mphutsi rumors as they were perceived as most likely to get the disease and suffer symptoms. If mphutsi rumors function as a revenge fantasy in any way then they feature as revenge against guilty women who lure hapless men.

Studies of AIDS contemporary legends in North America have shown that legends about deliberate infections tend to be the most popular and consistent (Goldstein, 2004: 46). Indeed, many aspects of observations made by Goldstein (citing the work of Joel Best) about

Western AIDS rumors and panics may easily apply to mphutsi rumors or other rumors circulating in Malawi featuring deliberate infection:

> The infector in these narratives has murderous intent, portrayed as a desire for random revenge. Generally, the attack is not directed at specific individuals, which makes the revenge even more frightening as it suggests that everyone is equally at risk... (Goldstein, 2004: 47)

In the case of mphutsi rumors strangers are targeted but not randomly as they are selected by gender (women) and profession (sex workers).

The most compelling interpretation of the mphutsi liver treatment and the quick time from infection to death revolves around the insecurity of the ARV supply chain. Malawi depends on foreign donors to fund the free ARV treatment programs. When bilateral, multilateral, or international NGO relationships sour and when bureaucratic and logistical coordination complexities multiple, medicine stock outs (shortages) occur, endangering the lives of those who rely on ARVs to prolong their lives. One particular telling of the mphutsi rumor (cited earlier) expresses this concern very poignantly. Emma Willard spoke of a woman who contracted mphutsi from a white lover and who then received money from that rich lover to treat the disease but died anyway. The belief that AIDS was brought from outsiders to Malawi is an obvious parallel. The current dependency of Malawi on foreign organizations or nations for treatments those outsiders can easily afford is another parallel. Mphutsi rumors suggest that at this point in the AIDS epidemic the optimism of seeing people live longer with AIDS is tempered by the fear that supply stock outs and capricious donors may threaten the fragile recovery experienced by Malawians and return the nation to the earlier reality of swift deaths wherein people have no "time to die." The very tenaciousness of HIV in the body, treated but not cured, adds to this persistent fear.

Conclusion

The story of AIDS in Malawi and sub-Saharan has an arc. In recent years, the narrative has moved from one of inevitable death for AIDS sufferers to one of tentative optimism in which people are raised from the brink of death to health with antiretroviral medicines. Some public health observers say that the tide has turned from ever increasing rates of new infections and high death rates to decreasing rates of new cases and a slowing of the AIDS death rates. Individuals in communities plagued by AIDS observe these changes, but they have also made changes. After three decades of living with AIDS, Malawians have modified their approaches to sexual relationships, changing the way they select partners and reducing the number of sexual partners they choose. All of these transformations may speak to a growing sense of AIDS being normalized as part of everyday life. The spirit and moment of acute crisis may have passed.

Yet, mphutsi rumors, articulate a contradiction. On one hand *mphusti* was described as a disease that was more dangerous that AIDS, kills more quickly than AIDS ever did, is more frighteningly visible and shameful than AIDS, and just as incurable. Mphutsi is more fire. It is worse than AIDS. Yet, at the same time it is AIDS. It is AIDS before ARVs; it is AIDS before the disease was seen as part of the general population. It is a disease that is too expensive to treat. It is a disease that strikes "at risk" people like sex workers. It is a disease brought by foreigners. And being like AIDS it is a disease with the potential to spread from the "at risk" to the general population. Mphutsi reawakens fears of the pre-ARV era just at a time when antiretrovirals have transformed the prospect of AIDS from inevitable death to chronic illness. Normalacy is mocked. But mphutsi is not only a vision of the past returned, it is also a fear for the present. Shortages of life prolonging AIDS medicines are a constant reminder that there is no cure for AIDS and that HIV resides stubbornly in the body. The whims of donors and bureaucracy stand between life and death for those receiving free ARVs.

Mphutsi rumors also reveal that questions of culpability have in no way faded from popular concern. Sex workers, identified early in the AIDS epidemic as "reservoirs" of disease, continue to serve as scapegoats. In a continuation of that legacy, sex workers in Lilongwe were attacked by men when mphutsi rumors were at their height. Mphutsi was described as a punishment for sex workers; women were described as extraordinarily vulnerable to both contracting mphutsi and also suffering from it. Vulnerability and suffering are not equally distributed between men and women. This may be linked to a sense of women's greater culpability in spreading disease by tempting helpless men into sexual liaisons.

The tendency to blame women for spreading disease can have significant consequences whether it results in attacks on sex workers and women wearing trousers or obscures the role of people not easily categorized as "prostitute" in transmitting diseases sexually. Rumors, like gossip, may be seen as a form of social control, implicitly or explicitly prescribing good behavior and sanctioning the bad, defining what is acceptable and what is unacceptable. Mphutsi rumors' very gendered nature are an obvious critique on "a certain type of woman," but they may also reveal concerns about women's rights. These stories sprang up not only at a time when AIDS is beginning to be subdued but also at a time when women's rights issues are being heavily and publically promoted by NGOS and governmental agencies alike. If we see mphutsi as part of a larger discourse about disciplining women then the context of women's rights advocacy in Malawi becomes relevant. In the past when women's rights have been extended or publically defended in Malawi, a concern with male loss of control of women's sexuality has arisen (Chanock, 1998).

The next chapter examines another set of rumors or urban legend in the light of women's rights law. Stories of magical rape circulating in Malawi, while on the surface are a critique of men who sexually violate women, they more subtly critique men and the law for being unable to recognize or deal with certain types of abuse in the domestic sphere.

CHAPTER 5

MGONEKO: MAGICAL RAPE, MEDIA PANIC, AND GENDER-BASED VIOLENCE

It was Spring of 2006 and I was in Northern Malawi taking a break from my round of interviews. I had been invited to attend a conference for students being held by a Christian student organization in a town about an hour from my research site. I accepted the invitation and sat in the back of a large auditorium filled with hundreds of teenagers and the kind of energy you get only by pulling together so many youthful people. The students were asked to fill out slips of paper with questions or issues they wanted to voice and have answered. One of the organization's leaders stood on stage with a microphone in hand ready to respond. Some of the questions related to religious perspectives on sexuality. One student wanted to know whether it was proper for women to wear trousers. "It depends," replied the leader on stage, "on the cultural context." Another student said that they were concerned about what had taken place in the Ekwendeni Girls Secondary School dormitories. According to media reports, the girls there had recently been attacked in their sleep by a witch or Satanist who through magic had sex with all of them. Was it possible that these girls could be infected with HIV by these magical, sexual predators? I sat with baited breath to hear how he would reassure the students. Instead the man told the student that it was unclear whether someone could be infected in this way. The reason, he said, is that when the young women wake in the morning they find some fluids there so perhaps, as we know HIV is spread through the exchange of fluids, there is some danger there. He moved on from that question after this equivocal response.

I was stunned by the story of a dormitory full of teenage girls being sexually assaulted *en masse* via magic. I wondered what had occurred to arouse this panic among the young women. Were there other such accounts of magical assaults and, if so, how might we interpret them? What do these stories say about women's sense of vulnerability? What do we need to know about "the cultural context" to make sense of these tales? To answer these questions, I began to look for related reports articles in Malawian newspapers and searched for similar stories in the gossip reports of my research assistants. Finally, in 2010, I took my investigations a step further and interviewed 53 men and women in Zomba, Mchinji, and Rumphi Districts about *mgoneko*. Mgoneko is traditional medicine used to make people fall into a deep sleep so that the one who administers the medicine can "do something bad" while the victim is unable to wake up. While the dictionary definition is generic and refers vaguely to "bad" deeds (Pass, 2004: 267), in the stories I collected the practice of mgoneko was closely associated with rape. Mgoneko was generally said to be used by men who, failing to gain sexual access to women they desired, resorted to the use of medicine obtained from traditional healers to have sex with them. The medicine enables men to magically enter a woman's home despite locked doors or presence of a husband in the bed next to her. Or else the mgoneko charms were said to make the victim or others around them helpless to struggle against their attacker or cry out.

While the definition provided above identifies some general features found in mgoneko stories, there exists significant variance in the tales that are well worth examining alongside some of the more standard features. These variations when juxtaposed testify to a sadly rich array of vulnerabilities for women, married and unmarried. In this chapter, I explore several major motifs of mgoneko magical rape stories, interpreting them in light of the media hype over domestic violence. In turn, the media hype may be partially a reaction to new laws created to protect women and children from domestic violence. Malawi's transition to multiparty democracy in 1994 (from a one-party system that prevailed from the time of Malawi's independence from Britain in 1964) coincided with Malawi's ratification of multiple international resolutions to mitigate gender inequality and to protect the rights of women. At the same time, Malawi's media was liberalized, opening the way for the emergence of new radio stations and newspapers that articulate a mandate of informing new citizens of their freedoms and rights (*ufulu*) and also of entertaining. Within the main period of my dissertation fieldwork (November 2005–July 2006) newspapers often publicized sensational, horrific, and sometimes supernatural tales of domestic violence and child molestation in the context of alarmingly high rates of HIV infection. The media, in a barrage of editorial pieces, crimes reports, and articles citing human rights activists or government officials, made the case that domestic violence is on the rise in Malawi and linked to high rates of AIDS prevalence among vulnerable wives and young women. I suggest that to understand mgoneko stories as they are currently told they must be placed in the context of the intense attention given to domestic violence by the media. These stories must be linked to communities' perceptions of government efforts to implement women's rights reforms. I argue that mgoneko rape stories participate in a discourse of moral panic over domestic violence in Malawi.

The concept of moral panic was articulated by Stanley Cohen in his seminal work *Folk Devils and Moral Panics* in which he described the process whereby the media of modern societies periodically generate episodes of panic (1972). Moral panics, arise when the media identifies and calls public attention to a condition, episode, person, or groups of persons that it portrays as a threat to societal values. The threat is presented by the media in a "stylized and stereotypical fashion." The media calls for the reactions of experts—"editors, bishops, politicians, and other right thinking people" who offer "diagnoses and solutions" (As quoted in Shevory (2004: 3)). Moral panics can be produced out of new phenomena or from long standing phenomena to which they suddenly draw extraordinary attention. Moral panics can sometimes pass away quickly or else have significant impact on public policy and collective perceptions. In many cases, moral panics arise around marginalized groups or fears of rising crime or threats to moral values (Shevory, 2004: 3). While they may revolve around truly emergent trends, on many occasions moral panics arise when there is no evidence of rising crime or "new" threats. Such is the power and reach of mass media in disseminating messages that "they can dredge up feelings of dread and shame as they reveal real or potential social disorder" (Shevory, 2004: 5). Shevory, who draws on the concept of moral panic in a study about AIDS scapegoating in American media, prefers the term "media panic" as it focuses on the media's role in creating moral panics.[1]

Mgoneko stories feature many intriguing motifs that could be the subject of analysis. This chapter, however, focuses primarily upon three variants of the mgoneko rape stories and the motifs expressed therein. The first variant speaks of women raped through mgoneko in their homes, sometimes while their husbands lie next to them. The second variant includes stories of girls in dormitories attacked en masse. Finally, I turn to the publicity storm that surrounded a group of men known as *nachipanti* (meaning one who wears only underpants) who operated in an area of the city of Blantyre. These men were believed to use magic to enter homes to rape women, suck the blood of women and children, and beat them (even to death), and to rob their homes.

In my analysis, I argue that young women's collective fantasies of magical rape are not so much dreams of an initiation into their lives as sexual beings, but rather they are being initiated into lives of violated sexuality. Indeed, media vilification of sexual abuse perpetuated by male teachers and traditional initiation practices involving sex highlight adolescence as a terrifying period for women. Mgoneko stories suggest that even adulthood and marriage fail to eliminate a woman's vulnerability; in mgoneko tales husbands are not able to stop men from magically raping their wives. Indeed, sometimes they are there when it is happening, unaware or helpless to do anything. The image may evoke not just helplessness but also complicity. This variant of the mgoneko genre may index the debate taking place in Malawi about whether women have the right to choose when they will and will not have sex with their spouses. The question of whether women have the right to refuse sex to their husbands has caused some concern among local communities as they seek to implement new women's rights policies. Thus women continue to find their homes and even their marriage beds sites of potential danger and violation. Finally, by analyzing *nachipanti* rumors we can get a sense of what people think about who is responsible for dealing with issues of sexual abuse.

Nightmares: Women Attacked in Their Own Beds

Descriptions of mgoneko attacks varied in detail but some of the repeated motifs across mgoneko stories included dreams about sex, the sensation of paralysis, vaginal discharge as evidence of a sexual encounter, the intrusion of a masked stranger in the home through a locked door, and uncertainty about the nature and consequences of mgoneko assaults. While on the surface these stories suggest women fear molestation from strangers, I suggest that the details of these stories hint at an additional source of fear, a fear of the danger in one's own home from the familiar. Analyzing mgoneko stories in the context of the media attention given to cases of brutalities enacted by husbands upon their wives and debates over whether women have the right under international human rights mandates to refuse sex to their husbands, points us away from women's fear of "stranger danger" to fear of more intimate partners.

One young man we interviewed, Charles Gama, told us his sister's story of mgoneko. It took place when he was visiting his sister (whom he described as a "spinster") where she lived at Malawi's lakeshore. His sister knew a man who was fond of her and was always trying to propose to her but she was not interested in him because she had someone else. That night when Gama was sleeping over at his sister's house he heard her scream around 1:00 a.m. He thought someone was attacking her and ran to her room to see what was happening. "She told me she felt some heaviness on top of her, yeah, just some heaviness but the door was closed and everything was in position; she explained that 'somebody very heavy was coming [and] lying on top of me and I was not very strong to resist him... but I don't know what happened—[it] was just like magic.'" She said that when she was dreaming she recognized the man as the one who was bothering her daily. According to Gama, she was checked at the hospital and was told that someone had been sleeping with her. (Charles Gama, Zomba, July 2, 2010)

A fifteen-year-old girl named Gladys told Mary Botha, one of my journal writers, a story of mgoneko that similarly featured a woman being paralyzed but in this case the woman was also put into a deep sleep. Gladys described mgoneko as "part and parcel of witchcraft, they magically break into buildings and they sleep with a woman." When asked by another young woman whether the victim wakes up during mgoneko Gladys replied

> It never happens [that a woman wakes during mgoneko sleep], maybe by the power of the Lord it may, but it is like Wizards have the magic that makes you sleep so deep that sometimes you find that you have wee wee-ed [urinated] on [the] bed. I don't know how. But sometimes you feel that wizards have come but you can't scream, you can't push or move any part of your body. So it's like they make you sleep and they do their thing... (Mary Botha research journal, Lubali, April 29, 2006)

Similarly, a woman we interviewed in Zomba told us, "Some people will dream like someone was on top of me" (Beatrice Ntaja, Zomba,

July 2, 2010). Whereas a man in Mchinji told us, "He [a person using mgoneko] will *kill people's feelings*[2] and then start doing what he wants with them and sometimes a woman will feel as if she is doing it with her husband" (Victor Ziwa, Mchinji, July 26, 2010). When she realizes and tries to wake up, the man is gone. Or as another woman in Mchinji District said, "[T]hey will do it without you noticing it." When this happens to a woman, "she is found with sperms in the night or she would be as if she was dreaming. Then she will be surprised to what is happening" (Alice Makwinja, Michinji, July 2010).

In some cases, the paralysis created by mgoneko medicine was said to not only affect female victims but also their husbands if they were present. Hastings Mkandawire, one of the journalers, introduces his conversation on mgoneko by first establishing the reputation of Joseph, the mgoneko user. Joseph was a local man known for going after the wives of other men. To overcome the disadvantages that his unattractive appearance and poverty caused him in securing women as sexual partners he resorted to magic. He was suspected of using love potions to get women. Mkandawire wrote that Joseph used to be popular with many of the married ladies because of his use of charms until it became rumored that he "used to change women from one to another" and was thereafter suspected of having AIDS. When the love potions began to fail, he resorted to another method. Mkandawire explained

> The need for him to sleep with women was still there, and he was now to work out another method to continue enjoying other people wives.

He went back to his herbalist who told him to start using another method.

> Instead of proposing and making good arrangements to have sex with women, Joseph decided to get different charms locally called (Mgoneko).
>
> He started sleeping with other people wives while the woman was fast asleep and while the husband was also fast asleep even if on the same bed.
>
> What happens in this method as we hear from those [who] know this method at least deeper is that a man who have those charms go to the house he wants to go that night and do all sorts of charms outside.

These charms force the wife and the husband to go into a deep sleep.

> Then the man after checking that the two and everybody in the home are asleep, enters into the house and do sleep with the wife (lady) he wants up to the end of the game. (Mkandawire research journal, Rumphi, July 2008)

In another incident involving mgoneko, also told by Mkandawire, it is the absence of the husband that makes it possible for "a mgoneko man" to take advantage of a woman. He writes

> Specifically the Mgoneko herb is meant for the people doing it [to] go into the targeted houses and sleep with the wife of that house without the owner [husband] noticing it. Even the woman being used doesn't exactly know what happens to her at the time of action. From reliable sources it is said that a victim—the woman—feels like [she is] in wet dreams when the Mgoneko man is really doing it. After the action, it is when the man discovers that she was sleeping with the mgoneko man. It is sad because it is said that the owner of the wife is forced to be away from the woman so that the mgoneko man should freely do his work. (Mkandawire research journal, Rumphi, November 14, 2008)

Erotic dreams are a common element in mgoneko stories, though not always central. A woman in Mchinji District (central Malawi) said that the way a woman knows that mgoneko has been used on her is because the man in the dream performs sex in a way that was not the norm for her husband. Afterwards when a woman wakes she finds "something strange," referring to a genital discharge in her underwear that is interpreted sometimes as semen. Another woman named Doreen, living in Zomba district in Southern Malawi, told us that she sometimes dreams that someone is sleeping with her and then wakes to find herself wet. She interpreted some of these occurrences as natural sex dreams but she said she used to have other dreams in which a tortoise would come to sleep with her. These tortoises, she said, were witches who came to amuse themselves with her. She had these dreams of tortoises on a regular basis until her mother gave her medicine to stop them from coming to the house. After getting the medicine she has stopped dreaming about them. She said that she never discovered who was doing these things to her because they came wearing a different face. Doreen's friend Bula said she had not experienced mgoneko herself but that her mother had when she was young. When Bula's mother was young she would dream that her uncle was sleeping with her and wake to find herself wet. She told her husband about it and they prayed over the matter. Later they came to the determination that she was being bewitched (Doreen Masamba and Bula Matola Zomba, July 3, 2010).

Interpreting Dreams and Stories about Dreams: Somatic Experiences and Cultural Context

How does one interpret dreams and, taking a step further, how does one interpret stories about dreams? The interpretation of dreams has been undertaken most famously by psychologist Sigmund Freud but dreams have also been the subject of interest to anthropologists, historians, and religious studies scholars. Generally speaking, all who study dreams have found some difficulty in disentangling the raw phenomenological experiences of the erotic dreams or nightmares from the cultural imagery and explanations for them. Part of this difficulty stems from the varieties of sources analyzed (some scholars consult firsthand accounts of dreams, nightmares, sleep paralysis, etc., while others draw upon oral traditions such as incubus, The Old Hag, witch riding, vampires, etc.). Another cause of difficulty in distinguishing experiences from cultural trappings stems from confusion in terminology. In this section, I highlight some ways that academics have analyzed the experience of nightmares, erotic dreams, and sleep paralysis as well as traditions associated with these experiences.

While some scholars have emphasized the experiential or phenomenological basis for supernatural assault traditions (most strikingly by folklorist David Hufford), others have focused on either the psychological or cultural grounding of reported phenomena (1982). The ubiquity of certain experiences outside the explicit cultural or linguistic framing suggests that experiences play a central role in the making of traditions. This has certainly been proven to be the case in Hufford's North American study of the "old hag" tradition. While those informants in Canada and the United States who were familiar with the "old hag" tradition spoke of being "hag ridden" at night by a spirit or demon sent to sit or ride atop them, others who had no notion of the tradition described essentially the same features of awakening (or having an experience while descending into a sleep state), hearing or seeing someone or something come into the room and approach the bed, the sensation of a weight pressing on the chest, the inability to move or cry out, and a sense of dread or fear. The Old Hag tradition appears to be related to hallucinations accompanying hypnogogic (relating to the state before one is fully asleep) or hympnopompic (relating to the state before one has fully awakened) stages of sleep coupled with sleep paralysis. Similar experiences have been reported worldwide and have various names and traditions associated with them. Researchers have found that worldwide about 5-30 percent of the general population (not only those diagnosed with sleep pathologies) report experiencing at least one episode of sleep paralysis (Dahlitz and Parkes, 1993). While some of the meaning attached to the experience clearly derives directly from the feelings aroused in the moment, cultural framing provides another layer of meaning. Despite the ubiquity of such experiences across the world and over time, the meaning of them and the framing of them can vary dramatically.

In the case of mgoneko, we see that a wide variety of experiences are put under the rubric of the term. The reported sensation of heaviness or a weight on the chest, the sense of some presence, the inability to move or resist that weight, and wakefulness is strongly suggestive of the kind of experience Hufford labels as sleep paralysis accompanied by hypnogogic hallucination (HH). While some accounts seem to suggest cultural framing of experiences of sleep paralysis and HH, other accounts of mgoneko do not include features of paralysis and wakefulness. Instead they speak of being in a deep sleep and having dreams about sexual intercourse. They speak specifically of waking in the morning to find genital discharge but not having any awareness of being violated as they slept. What can we make of this? In analyzing these stories and trying to fit the reported episodes of mgoneko into insights into physiological aspects of the sleep cycle, I must proceed with caution. While Hufford devised his research methods to identify characteristic phenomenological patterning of observations and sensations, my sources of information about mgoneko include neither his systematic probing of perceptions nor such a large sample. Thus any connection I make between patterns in mgoneko story motifs to insights into phases of sleep must be taken as suggestive rather than conclusive. That being said I suggest that what is called mgoneko may be related to a variety of distinct phases of sleep phenomena. As mentioned above some mgoneko tales suggest the experience of HHs. Other aspects of mgoneko seem akin to sleep paralysis with accompanying sense of dread or fear. Such experiences may play a significant role in the development of the tradition. Other accounts of mgoneko do not seem to involve paralysis or inspire dread but rather may be categorized as erotic dreams accompanied by nocturnal emissions (wet dreams). Though sleep paralysis with hallucinations and erotic dreams are physiologically distinct in nature, in Malawi these two types of experiences are interpreted similarly.

The interpretation of somatic experiences can vary widely depending on cultural context as aptly demonstrated by Charles Stewart in his analysis of what he calls "erotic nightmares" in the European context. The erotic dream is defined by Stewart as a dream with erotic content, which may or may not be accompanied by sexual stimulation, "nocturnal emissions," and orgasm. Though these erotic dreams have been unwelcome in some epochs, they have sometimes been unwelcome because their content is pleasurable and suggests lack of self-control. The nightmare, by contrast, has been deemed undesirable for different reasons; the classic nightmare involves "dream visions where the sleeper feels a weight on his or her chest and has accompanying sensation of dyspnoea [difficulty breathing or catching one's breath], paralysis, and dread (Stewart, 2002: 282)." European terminology for nightmares register beliefs about a demonic presence that sits on, presses, or strangles people as they sleep. Over time the erotic dream and the nightmare were fused in European societies and then later delinked.

For some time the erotic dream and the nightmare seemed to be categorized as separate types of experiences in ancient Greece. However, by the first century CE in Greece, there is some linguistic evidence that descriptions of the nightmare had begun to take on sexual connotations. Stewart points to the probable influence of the Roman imperial regime and the growing influence of Christianity.

> In rendering the [Greek word for nightmare] idea of "jumping upon" into Latin, however, the translators enmeshed in a matrix of words that contained clear sexual connotations—for example *concumbere* "to sleep (with)" and *concubinus* "concubine." (Stewart, 2002: 286)

Beyond attributing this shift in ideas to "semantic contagion," Stewart identifies the influence of Stoics' notion of self-regulation and moderation as well as the influence of Christian ascetics. This is not to say that previous to these developments no one in Greece experienced erotic nightmares but that there was no focus on or vocabulary for it.

Both linguistic borrowing and the evolution of ideas of self-hood lead to particular formulations of the erotic nightmares over time.

Mgoneko accounts vary from having a close similarity to the non-sexual, oppressive nightmare in which a person feels a weight on the chest, has difficulty moving and breathing, and feels a strong sense of dread to the erotic dream that does not strike the dreamer as problematic until they reflect upon it in the morning. From accounts of mgoneko erotic dreams one might surmise that the dreams are pleasurable as the women say they feel as if they are having sex and sometimes believe it is their husbands with whom they are having sex. Without an explicit description of violence or alarm expressed, we may assume that these dreams lack that sense of dread associated with the "classic nightmare" and may actually be pleasurable. What is striking in most descriptions of the mgoneko attacks is how in those which seem to be erotic dreams, fear and concern rests in the non-consensual nature of mgoneko sex. Gama's sister was upset about the mgoneko incident mostly because she had rejected the advances of the man she blamed for her troubling dream. It is his insistence on having sex with her through the sneaking, troublesome, and illegitimate manner despite her refusal that is most alarming. An excerpt from another journal entry serves to emphasize this point. A young woman named Goodness relates a story about a woman who used medicines [described as "charms"] to stop men from using mgoneko on her. In this case, the medicine did not so much stop such incidents from occurring but allowed it to be revealed to her:

> Goodness: I have my own story to tell and this happened to Isazo... So what happened was that sister Isazo was charmed [so] that no one would perform any kind of witchcraft on her. One thing that kept men's eyes on her was her beauty and attraction. Many men even married ones were proposing her but no one succeeded. Up to that [time when she started using the protective medicine] some were coming at night so that they should just perform the Mgoneko on her. And every time that they would come she would tell me.
>
> One night there came a man who told [her] that he will come to see [her]. She thought that the man would come normally. In the night, Isazo woke up and the man found her awake. She told him that she was not one so foolish. Now what happened was that we went to a grocery to buy tea leaves and we [ran] into him and she was like, "You are the [one] I'm looking for, what did you want from me in the night when you came? I warn you, that was the second time! Am I lying?" and the

> man answered "No!" I tell you the woman shouted at the man up to the point that the man feared her and told her in the face that you are dangerous. Later in the evening she told [me] about the charm. (Mary Botha research journal, Lubali, April 29, 2006)

Women's expressions of outrage and fear upon waking from an mgoneko incident juxtaposed with the feeling of paralysis or being put into a deep sleep expose women's loss of control and forced submission. That women are in a deep sleep is a further dramatization of their vulnerability when it comes to issues of sexual agency. I say "women" generally because I was told by my informants that it was almost always men who performed mgoneko on women and not the other way around. Some were not sure that a woman could even "mgoneko" man. Does this mean that men do not have erotic dreams? This is highly unlikely as erotic dreams appear to be a universal phenomenon. What one may conclude rather is that Malawian culture encourages divergent interpretations of men's erotic dreams versus women's erotic dreams. While some erotic dreams may appear to be "naturally occurring," others strike the dreamer as unwelcome with respect to the partner or nature of consent. How are dreams interpreted in Malawi? What relationship is the waking world believed to have with the dream life?

In Malawi, people interpret dreams in several ways. Some dreams are viewed as ordinary, not particularly meaningful, reflecting waking thoughts, desires, and concerns. However, in dreams one has the opportunity to come in closer contact to the spiritual realm. Some dreams are said to carry messages from spirits, particularly ancestors. For example, a dream communication with a deceased elder is usually the means by which diviner healers come into their vocations, learn about medicines, and receive guidance. Some dreams are considered prophetic and the dreamer has the burden of sharing the message with others (e.g., Friedson (1996: 9-37) and Schoffeleers (1999: 407-409)). However, dreams can be invaded by troublesome spirits such a witches and their familiars. The meddling of witches with the sleeping is believed to cause sleeplessness and sickness. Thus some dreams are believed to have special significance in the waking, material realm such that there is no unambiguous ontological distinction made between the waking and sleeping world. Such beliefs regarding dreams are present throughout Central and Southern Africa (see Schoffeleers (1999: 409)). The ambiguous relationship between the sleeping and waking world helps account for the fear that some express with regards to mgoneko.

Oral traditions about people who trouble the sleeping or unconscious include those told in Central and East Central Africa about blood suckers (variously called *mumiami*, *banyama*, *chifwamba*, vampires, *wazi-mamoto*, *kuchinja*, etc.) who were sometimes said to cause their victims to become "dull," powerless, and unable to cry out. During the colonial period bloodsuckers were said to be African agents of European colonial governments who captured other Africans and made them unconscious by administering some type of drug in order to drain their blood. The blood was then given to Europeans to enhance their own health. Like mgoneko stories these tales include a motif of being made helpless and vulnerable through the use of medicine and like mgoneko tales they are also gendered. According to Luise White, males spoke of being made dull or impotent while women spoke of having their mouths bandaged and being unable to shout or talk (White, 2000: 117). White analyzes these elements as reflective of specific colonial medical practices involving anesthesia. Though presumably putting people to sleep was meant as a step toward treatment and healing, the popular stories arising from them suggests African subjects read more nefarious purposes and possibilities in these treatments. Women in particular seemed to feel vulnerable to voicelessness in colonial regimes (White, 2000:120). Women's sense of vulnerability seems to have extended into the current postcolonial era.

In Southern Africa (particularly Zimbabwe and South Africa), stories circulate about troublesome creatures known as the *thikoloshe*. *Thikoloshe* are described as half child-like and half ape-like creatures that are hairy, have one buttock, and large sexual organs. These days *thikoloshe* are said to be under the control of witches. They are thieves who also attempt to have sex with women as they sleep. In the past, women would elevate their beds to keep *thikoloshe* from climbing in the bed to rape them. *Thikoloshe* are seen as nasty and harmful but rarely causing death (Bahre, 2002). Indeed, sometimes stories about them provoke laughter. Mgoneko tales certainly seem to share some elements with *thikoloshe* stories (i.e., supernatural beings who assail women at night), however, it is not my aim here to discover the precise nature of that relationship but rather to simply point out some of the imagery and ideas circulating regionally, which may account for the interpretation of certain dreams or sleep paralysis episodes in Malawi. Like stories of men who use mgoneko, *thikoloshe* stories are not always about suppressed or repressed sexual desire. While on one hand mgoneko and *thikoloshe* stories may represent the desires of men who have difficulty fulfilling sexual needs and women who desire illicit, extramarital sex, on the other hand they represent anxieties about sex. Several scholars have pointed out how *thikoloshe* or other familiars have represented fear about rape or expressed women's dissatisfaction with their sexual roles in marriage (see Bahre's discussion of Lee (1969) and Hammond-Tooke (1974) in Bahre (2002: 327-328)). Malawian women may also be expressing their concerns about their sexual roles in marriage when they tell stories about mgoneko men.

Women's Right to Refuse Sex and the Controversy over Marital Rape

A number of policies for strengthening women's rights in Malawi have been instituted in the last few decades. In 1987, Malawi ratified the UN's Convention on the Elimination of All Forms of Discrimination Against Women. In 1993, the Women in Development strategy for incorporating women's concerns into development projects was adopted. The 1995, the Constitution of the Republic of Malawi made achieving gender equality a constitutional principle. In 2006, Malawi adopted new policies to better guard women against domestic violence by ratifying The Prevention of Domestic Violence Act. Malawi has a National Gender Policy and an agency specifically charged with formulating, implementing, coordinating, monitoring, and evaluating gender policy. In addition to government efforts, NGOs operating in Malawi urge changes in government policies and the attitudes/behavior of the general public.

The Women and Law in Southern Africa Research and Educational Trust (WLSA) made efforts in 2001 to get federal legislation to recognize and criminalize marital rape. As the law stands, rape in Malawi is defined as forcing a member of the opposite sex who is not one's spouse to have sex. WLSA's stance on marital rape is controversial in Malawi. One Supreme Court Justice said such a law is not consistent to the continued existence of marriage because, "[b]y entering into marriage each spouse is taken to have consented to sexual intercourse." Seodi White, Malawi's National Coordinator of WLSA in Malawi, rebuts that 75 percent of Malawian women have been forced to have sex with a husband who has come home drunk or drugged or have been raped as a means of punishment. (*BBC News*, Row over Malawi marital rape bill, December 26, 2001).[3] Media sources magnified the controversy by portraying local leaders (village headmen, elder, chiefs, church leaders, governmental officials, men in general) as resistant to enforcing women's rights laws because as husbands men had the right to sex with their wives when they wanted. When a prominent Malawi newspaper asked one man about women's right to refuse sex to husbands, the man predicted "...this right will bring death" (*The Nation*, February 27, 2006). Men and women whose comments were featured in the article said that refusing sex to a husband was a form of gender violence that forced men to seek sexual partners outside marriage where they risked contracting HIV and visiting the disease upon the whole family.

> "...if a woman refuses to sleep with her husband, she puts the family at a risk as a man would go for other women and contract HIV and Aids. If you give a woman the right to say no to sex with her husband, you are at the same time giving the man the right to have sex outside the marriage. And this right will bring death in the family through HIV and Aids." (*The Nation*, Refusing sex is gender-based violence, February 27, 2006)

Initially I suspected that the authors of such newspaper articles, who are part of Malawi's educated elite, were not-so-subtly mocking the "ignorant" and "uncivilized" villagers. However, in 2010, similar sentiments were echoed in my interviews with several village elders in Rumphi who were in charge of implementing women's rights policies locally.

In that same village I interviewed individuals involved in Lekani Nkhanza (meaning "stop violence"), an organization funded by the German aid agency, GTZ, that partnered with the government of Malawi to educate people about women's rights and train local intermediaries to intervene in cases involving domestic violence. I asked them what challenges they faced in carrying out these objectives. I was told by the respondents that there is a need to adapt international policies to Malawian cultural values. In particular, I was told that the framing of international language on women's rights failed to take into account men's rights in wives and wives' responsibilities. It was feared that women would try to take advantage of their newly protected rights by refusing sex to their husbands without acceptable, customary justifications for abstinence (sickness, pregnancy, menstruation, when a woman is nursing, and other periods requiring ritual abstinence). I followed up such discourse by asking if there was any concern about men denying women sex. Some of my respondents found this question laughable (I say this because several literally laughed). One opining that men will always want sex and that if a wife wants sex he will feel lucky and always say yes (Victor Ziwa Mchinji, July 26, 2010). In other words, there was no danger of men refusing sex to women but only the reverse. This perception, however, was false in that a common complaint made by women in polygamous marriages arises from the refusal of a man to sleep with one of his wives in favor of another. However, the few men I mentioned this to forgot about this common complaint until I brought it up. What is important is that there is a perception and fear that women will capriciously refuse sex to husbands despite their obligations.

A Freudian reading of mgoneko stories might suggest that mgoneko dreams are a wish fulfillment of women, that they represent women's suppressed or repressed desire to have sex with men other than their husbands (Freud 1950). One informant said that women may think that during an mgoneko incident they are having sex with their husbands until they realize that the man performs sex in an unfamiliar way. The unfamiliar might be welcome. I can make no claims of having probed the subconscious desires of women and instead examine people's conscious interpretations and their collective framing of mgoneko. The horror women express and the actions they take in seeking redress and finding medicine to protect themselves from future attacks frames mgoneko as not a part of women's fantasy genre but rather as a horror story, a collective nightmare. While it is impossible to gauge the prevalence of concern about women insisting on a right to refuse sex to husbands based on a few anecdotes, mgoneko stories point to well-publicized stories of domestic violence. Mgoneko tales suggestively combine elements of sexual violence committed by familiar culprits in domestic settings. If mgoneko is a woman's nightmare what analog does it have in everyday life? Do women fear sexual assaults from strangers?

Possibly, but the venue of mgoneko attacks points to domestically situated "gender-based violence," (GBV) the term preferred by multilateral organizations, state officials, and nongovernmental agencies in Malawi to refer to a broad range of physically, emotionally, financially, and/or socially coercive actions by which women are controlled by elders or males with whom they are intimately connected (NSO,

2011: 239). Sexual assault is only one form of women's insecurity in their own homes. Statistics on violence against women in Malawi bear out that most physical violence against women (as everywhere else in the world) is perpetuated in intimate relationships rather than by strangers. About 70 percent of women aged 15-49 who had experienced gender-based violence since the age of 15 had been victimized by either a current or former spouse or boyfriend. Another 24 percent had suffered at the hands of relatives (NSO, 2011: 242). Most danger comes from within a family. In 2006, Malawi adopted new policies to protect women against violence in the domestic sphere including the creation of protective orders (restraining orders) and occupancy orders (that grant a woman to the right to remain in the marital home but prohibits her abuser from returning until the order is reversed). In addition, police units known as Victim Support Units (VSU) were created in 2001 as part of a community policing initiative. They are trained to help counsel women as to their rights, assist in prosecutions, and sometimes provide temporary shelter. Meanwhile, the media ran a series of sensational stories about domestic violence and child molestation.

Media and Gender-Based Violence

The flipside of men's concern with women using their human rights to refuse sex is women's concern with their difficulties in refusing sex. The 2010 Malawi Demographic and Health Survey (MDHS) reported that of Ever-Married Women about 19 percent of women aged 15-49 reported having experienced sexual violence at least once with their husband or current partner. Sexual violence in this survey was defined as being physically forced to have intercourse when one does not want to or being forced to perform sexual acts that one does not want to perform. Of women who have ever been married about 13 percent said they experienced sexual violence "often or sometimes" (NSO, 2011: 250). While the pervasiveness of the experience creates one level of awareness in communities, the media adds another level. In 2005 and 2006, while I was conducting my dissertation research issues of rape, domestic violence, and child molestation garnered significant and persistent coverage in the newspapers and on the radio airwaves.

Indeed the media may have stirred a panic by consistently linking gender-based violence, HIV/AIDS and human rights. When I say that media linked these issues I do not mean to say that this was done illegitimately but rather to highlight the power of the media in bringing together three highly charged areas of anxiety for the public. From November 2005 through April 2006 I monitored the print media, primarily the most circulated newspapers—*The Nation* and *The Daily Times*. I also worked with two assistants who monitored and reported on AIDS-related radio broadcasts in Rumphi District. I found that a "media panic" was stirred up through sensational narratives and images, processes of repetition, claims made by various experts (including the journalists themselves), the linkages the media articulated between events and concepts, and finally, through pointed critiques of dysfunctional aspects of society.

One of the most memorable stories was that of a woman in Central Malawi in the Dowa district who was attacked by the man she had recently divorced. Marrieta Samuel had decided to divorce her husband Herbert Mankhwala despite the efforts of marriage counselors to keep the marriage together. In January 2007, he lay in wait for her among the high maize stalks and attacked her with a panga knife (machete) chopping both her arms such that the hospital had to amputate them both below the elbow. When interviewed later Mankhwala claimed that he had been driven to rage after discovering his ex-wife "committing adultery" with the owner of the maize field where he had attacked Samuel. After spying on the couple Mankhwala dashed home to find a knife and returned to the field to attack his ex-wife. In reaction to the event, the then Malawian Minister of Gender, Child Welfare, and Community Services Joyce Banda said, "it was disturbing to note that incidents of inhuman treatments perpetuated to vulnerable women and children were rampant" (*The Nation*, Husband chops wife's arms, January 10, 2006).

The same month in the Northern district of Karonga a man was accused of killing his wife after she refused to have sex with him. A police spokesperson was quoted saying, "'Simbeye wanted to have sex with his wife, Leah Nyahunga at around 8 o'clock in the evening but she refused, saying they could not do that since they are HIV positive. Her refusal angered the man who beat her,' he alleged." (*The Nation*, Man kills wife after refusing sex, January 11, 2006). And again in January 2006 in the Southern district of Thyolo a 31-year-old man was arrested for killing his wife and child. A Blantyre police official claimed the man was angry that his wife continued to work for a certain company despite his disapproval. After she went to stay with her family to continue working for her employer her husband attacked her, stabbing her in the neck, back, and ribs and then running away. Her neighbours eventually found her body in the house and later her husband surrendered to the police. He confessed that he also killed their child whom he then stowed in a travel bag. The newspaper reported, "The deaths come in the wake of many reports of women abuse[d] by men recently."

The chopping incident in conjunction with other high-profile cases of the time came to exemplify what was wrong with gender relations in Malawi. The Director of Women's Affairs for the Democratic Progressive Party Patricia Kaliati and Malawi's president Bingu wa Mutharika presented the three-months pregnant Marietta Samuel with money. Kaliati and other members of the DPP (pictured in Figure 5.1) visited Samuel in the hospital to comfort her. According to *The Nation* Kaliati remarked that violence against women was rampant in Malawi and continued by lauding the efforts of human rights

Hacking victim gets K100,000 from Bingu

'She's 3 months pregnant'

by James Chimpweya

President Bingu wa Mutharika on Sunday gave K100,000 to 31-year-old Marietta Samuel who had both her arms chopped off by her estranged husband Herbert Mankhwala two weeks ago.

Democratic Progressive Party (DPP) Director of Women Affairs Patricia Kaliati said Mutharika was shocked to learn that Samuel had her arms chopped by her estranged husband.

Kaliati said Mutharika decided to give her K100,000 to enable her do some small businesses after being discharged from the hospital.

Kaliati, who is also Information and Tourism Minister, gave Samuel the money at Kamuzu Central Hospital (KCH) in Lilongwe where DPP women went to cheer and pray for the victim.

The prayer of comfort was given by Kaliati herself who asked God to intervene on violence against women which, she said, is rampant in the country.

Kaliati also applauded human rights activists who, she said, were doing a commendable job in dealing and sensitising people on gender violence against women and appealed to men to lend them an ear.

"Sex should be done when the two parties have agreed and one should not be forced because we are all daughters and sons of one God. Men should regard us as partners in marriage and treat us humanely," she said.

She said Mutharika's donation would be deposited in a bank in Dowa today for Samuel to use after being discharged.

Lucy Mkutumula, KCH Principal Nursing Officer, said Samuel's condition was now improving.

"When she came here she lost a lot of blood but now she is improving tremendously. She is now able to sit which she was failing when she was being admitted," said Mkutumula, adding that Samuel is three months pregnant.

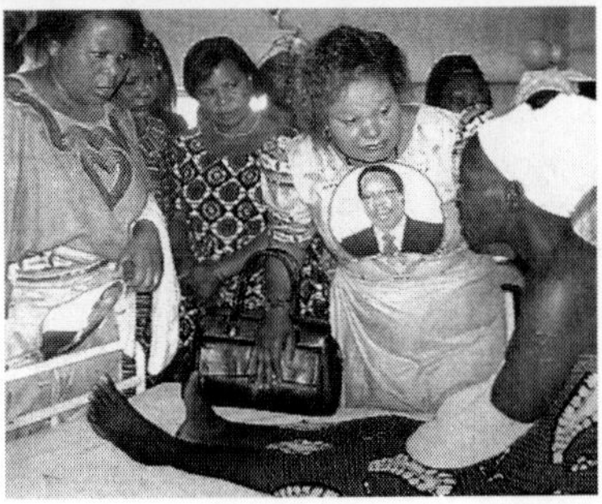

Get well soon: Kaliati (2nd R) and other DPP women cheering Samuel (R).—*Pic: James Chimpweya*

Samuel's mother, Dezideleta Katema, said her daughter had seven cuts in the head.

Meanwhile, the estranged husband is still at large.

During the visit, Kaliati said, DPP women also donated K30,000 part of which would be given to a poor woman who gave birth to triplets at the Bottom Hospital in Lilongwe two weeks ago. She said the other amount would be given to other vulnerable patients at Kamuzu Central Hospital.

Figure 5.1 Courtesy of Nation Publications Ltd, Newspaper article with photograph entitled "Hacking Victim gets K100,000 from Bingu." *The Nation*. Jan. 17, 2006.

activists in "sensitizing people on gender violence against women and appealed to men to lend them an ear. 'Sex should be done when the two parties have agreed and one should not be forced because we are all daughters and sons of one God. Men should regard us as partners in marriage and treat us humanely, she [Kaliati] said.'" (*The Nation*, Hacking victim gets K100,000 from Bingu: She's 3 months pregnant, January 17, 2006)

Yet it was not just human rights activists "sensitizing" people to the evils of gender-based violence, the media may also play a major role in heightening the sense of urgency around the topic. By returning to the same narrative frequently, the media created an impression of high and rising prevalence of domestic violence. The list of headlines from *The Nation* below chronicle a steady stream of reporting on GBV and child molestation:

July 18, 2005 Gender based violence on the increase

July 25, 2005 Defiler gets 8 years IHL [Imprisonment with Hard Labor]

Aug. 10, 2005 Teacher arrested for suspected rape

Nov. 11, 2005 Girl, 13, defiled, forced to abort

Nov. 11, 2005 Silence fueling incest

Nov. 25, 2005 Teacher gets six years for defiling own pupil

Nov. 28, 2005 LL [Lilongwe] Man arrested for defiling 4 months old baby

Dec. 3, 2005 Sex with 4 month old babies

Dec. 8, 2005 Man gets 8 years for defiling baby

Dec. 12, 2005 Something is terribly wrong

Dec. 14, 2005 Deal with rapists—Letters

Dec. 15, 2005 Zabweka: I'm in for the offence of molesting a two months old baby" (Zabweka is a satirical cartoon)

In January 2006, the media's attention shifted from an emphasis on the sexual molestation of children or teenage girls to an emphasis on men beating their wives. The incident in Dowa in which Samuel's arms were chopped marked this turning point. Below is a sample of relevant headlines from *The Nation*:

Jan. 10 Husband chops wife's arms

Jan. 11 Man kills wife after refusing sex

Jan. 18 On molestation, wife battering

Jan. 21 HRCC condemns gender based violence

Jan. 23 Man kills wife, child

Jan. 23 Any normal men left?—Letters

Jan. 24 Govt proposes bill to curb domestic violence

Jan. 24 Increased cases of violence sickening

Jan. 24 Man burns wife, himself

Jan. 24 Man in for infecting girl 14 with HIV

Jan. 24 The seamy side of our society

From *The Daily Times*:

Jan. 24 Man mutilates woman's private parts

Jan. 24 Man petrol bombs wife

Through constant repetition—with little variation on the theme—the media portrayed the sense that gender-based violence and child molestation in Malawi were occurring with increasing frequency. The media presented no statistical evidence that there had been a measurable increase in violent crimes against children and women beyond the sensationally brutal anecdotes and quotes by officials alarmed by the increasing *reports* of violence. At the center of these media reports of domestic violence were women's refusals to consent to sex with their husbands or submit in some other way to their husbands' wishes. One edition of *Zabweka*, a cartoon serial run in *The Nation* featuring the misadventures of a lecherous middle-aged man, plays with the questions about women's rights and men's violence. In the cartoon (Figure 5.2) Zabweka is holding a panga knife in one hand and reaching for a woman's throat with the other. A male bystander intervenes by saying that the woman's refusal to shake Zabweka's hand was not sufficient grounds to grant him the right to chop off her hands.

In a sense the cartoon simultaneously illustrates a problem and one of its solution as formulated by government officials and nongovernmental human rights activists. The problem is that men violate women's rights through violence when women exercise their rights to refuse sex or defy men in some other manner; the solution is for other men to intervene and make the abuse of women their own problem rather than stand by idly.

How do the narratives and images circulating in media relate to mgoneko beliefs? It poses some problems to simply assert that

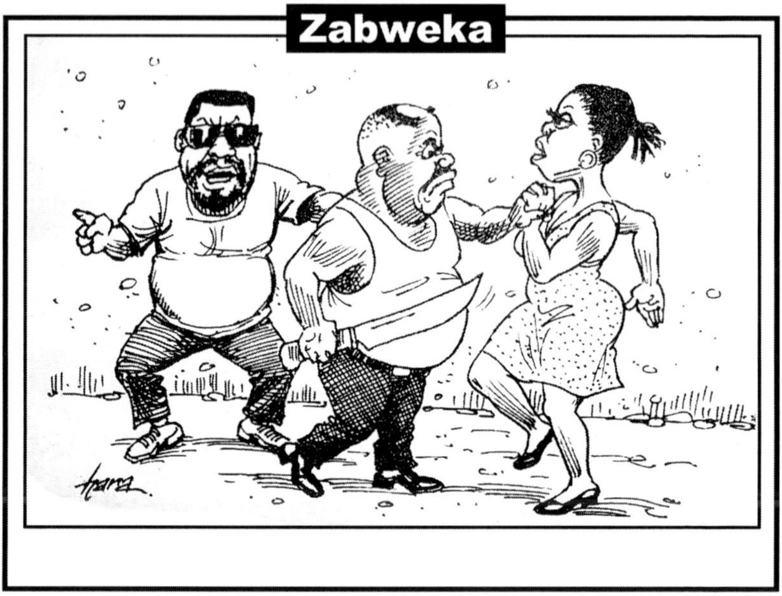

Figure 5.2 Courtesy of Nation Publications Ltd, "Leave her alone, will you? The fact that she refused to give you a handshake does not give you any right to chop off her hands!" By Brian Hara in *The Nation,* Mar 11–12, 2006.

mgoneko stories are about intimate partner violence as the culprits in these stories are emphatically identified as not husbands or boyfriends but rather as other, albeit familiar men in the community. Indeed, one might say that mgoneko stories reverse the roles that husbands and strangers typically play in the everyday waking world of gender-based violence. In everyday life husbands and boyfriends are responsible for perpetuating the overwhelming majority of sexual abuse and battery. What can we say then about this role reversal? What does it tell about the meaning of mgoneko stories? Part of the popularity of mgoneko tales (and rumors generally) derives from their shock value. Gossip, circulating within constrained social networks, is said to expose contradictions while rumor, circulating in broader context is described as explaining contradictions (White, 2000: 60). Gossip and rumor explore the violation of norms and linger on shocking inversions of proper social behaviors. At the same time rumors are not a complete inversions but should bare some resemblance to order of the world to have some intelligibility, relatability, and plausibility to the listeners. By saying that mgoneko stories point to domestic violence am I making them say something they do not say? Am I simply reversing the meaning they have for those who tell them? I think not. I argue that in the context of widespread and public debates about women's right to refuse sex, shocking and well publicized spousal abuse, the setting of the stories (home and bedroom behind locked doors) suggest a anxiety over the pervasiveness of intimate partner violence. A critique of domestic violence cannot be discarded even if the perpetrators in mgoneko tales are masked as strangers, especially if the perpetrator is a man wearing the guise of a husband.

Meanings in rumor and gossip are not singular or reducible. Another reading of mgoneko tales with respect to domestic violence can be formulated by asking why sexual coercion in the home is masked as "stranger danger?" Why is the role of the stranger and the husband reversed? One possibility is that by transforming intimate partner violence into violence from a stranger the problem of sexual abuse becomes a problem for more people in the community, both men and women. One hint of this was displayed in the village in Mchinji where all the women were said to have been magically assaulted by two or three men using witchcraft charms. In this case, some women said they were having dreams of sex while others did not have dreams. There was debate as to whether mgoneko sex could transmit HIV but no consensus. One woman we interviewed said that despite not having a mgoneko dream she went to get a blood test just in case. Both men and women in the community became angry and sought to have the alleged culprits punished. According to some we interviewed in that village, one of the mgoneko men was imprisoned for a year after being tried in a government court. One woman said that many people attended the trial and shouted at the man. The nature of the charge is unclear as it is against the law in Malawi to accuse someone of witchcraft.[4]

Beyond the concern a husband has for a wife's safety and security, he also has legal rights in his wife. A man who has sex with another man's wife is by custom violating not only that woman's rights but also her husband's rights. Traditionally a wronged husband can pursue compensatory damages from such a man through negotiations whether the sex act was consensual or an act of rape (Chanock, 1998: 192-216. See especially p. 197 for information about damages and rape.). In the realm of magical rape, any man can be wronged by an mgoneko man by no fault of their wives. In the case of the Mchinji village where men confessed to magically sleeping with all the women of a village all the husbands there had a stake in case. They had all been wronged. Mgoneko tales cleverly express the pervasive experience of the abuse of women's "new" rights (protection from gender-based violence) and aligns them with "traditional" rights of husbands thus serving a vital function of rumor—bringing together seeming contradictions.

AIDS, Human Rights, and Sexual Assault: Critical Linkages

The media play a role in connecting separate events to articulate the existence of a pervasive phenomenon. They also conceptually link phenomena to extralocal politics, social movements, and conflicts. In Malawi, the media narratively link the AIDS epidemic to what is described by their informants as an epidemic of rape. There is some evidence that the correlation is adopted by the public that consumes these narratives. One journaler, a woman in her early twenties, had the below conversation about rape and AIDS while traveling in a car with the colleagues she works with at a youth program. The journaler writes

> *The story [being broadcast on the radio in the car] was about one patient suffering from AIDS. She's a girl aged 22. She got the disease apparently because she was raped—that was in Lilongwe when she was staying with her aunt who died later 2004.*
>
> Mrs. Muwowo: I think the government has to do something about these rapists. Because many girls who are being found HIV positive nowadays you find out that they were raped. And I think nowadays raping doesn't only breach ones human rights but it can also be equated to murder. [Mrs. Muwowo went on to describe the way in which the girl was raped and another woman Ms. Lombe commented.]
>
> Ms. Lombe: That's very sad for a person to be found in that situation. I think there must be some stiff penalties for those who rape. I listened to Wings of Hope [a religious radio program featuring dramatizations] one of the Sundays—must be February this year—there was that interview with Reine Charity Ngozo the one in the NAC [Malawi National AIDS Commission] newsletter. She explained how she got the virus and it was that her own boyfriend raped her... And last week it was about Phinda Mughogho who was raped by a friend of her aunt. She fell sick and was later found HIV positive. There are more stories about girls who get infected about [by] being raped so I

> think this is getting more and more serious... (Mary Botha research journal, Rumphi, May 2, 2006)

In the same way, the women quoted above connected various isolated events, the media also connects isolated events, helping to create the impression that there is a trend. In newspapers, for example, instead of allowing each case to stand alone, reports of one crime were often tagged at the end with a "related story," the report of another similar, violent act. This practice helps foster the notion that some common social pathology undergirds all the incidents. In an article that begins with the words "[a]nother gruesome murder" a reporter describes an incident in which a man stabs his wife to death and then stomps on his toddler daughter also killing her. At the end of the article the reporter notes the increasing government attention to domestic violence and includes three "related stories":

> A woman from Dowa is recovering at Kamuzu Central Hospital after her husband chopped both her arms after she had denounced their marriage.
>
> Police are yet to arrest the husband.
>
> Another woman was beaten to death in Karonga by her husband after she refused him sex and a 60-year-old woman from Kasungu almost lost her sight after being attacked by two men.
>
> Secretary for Gender Andrina Mchiela is on record as saying government was doing everything possible to put mechanisms in place to check violence.
>
> Mchiela said the frequency of attacks on women this month raises a lot of suspicion to the effect that "one is forced to believe these gruesome acts are being carried through an organized syndicate." (*The Daily Times*, Hubby murders wife, daughter, January 23, 2006)

Besides relating disparate incidents, the media conceptually lump together cases of spousal abuse, incest, child molestation, and rape to form a general sense of increased violence against vulnerable segments of the population. In addition, the media consistently links gender-based violence with a risk of HIV infection for women. They assert—usually indirectly through those they interview or through the publication of opinion pieces—that violence or the threat of violence by husbands, expose women to a risk of HIV infection in their marriage beds. These discussions of rights husbands have over wives and rights women have over their own bodies spill over into discussions of "human rights":

> Elias Chakwera [then principal of the Domasi College of Education in Malawi], said gender and HIV and AIDS are two cross-cutting issues which need to be tackled together. "Gender has a stake in HIV and AIDS in that if you look at the population of people who are affected by the pandemic, the majority are girls. We feel that if we are to effectively combat the spread of the pandemic, women need to be empowered so that they can make informed choices regarding their sexual life." (*The Weekend Nation*, Linking gender to HIV and AIDS, July 9-10, 2005)

Another newspaper article provocatively entitled 'Wives at risk in their own beds" (*The Nation*, April 16, 2006) features the Parliamentary Committee on HIV/AIDS stating that women lack empowerment in the bedroom as well as in other aspects of their relationships with husbands. This, he says, is instilled in women during their initiations where they are taught to respect and obey their husbands. He concludes that women cannot question the movements and habits of their husbands (referencing extramarital sex) and therefore they risk exposure to HIV/AIDS in their own bedrooms. The media is playing a role in publicizing issues of domestic violence but also in relating linkages between human rights abuses, HIV/AIDS, and domestic violence. The question remains, however, what the role of "sensitization" will play in the lives of women who need empowerment.

Coming of Age: Dorm Room Initiations

The media, human rights agencies, and government ministries see themselves as taking an active role in empowering women through information. Yet they also expose scenarios that undercut the idea of women making "informed choices regarding their sexual lives." The stories featured in the news about young school girls preyed upon by older men, sometimes teachers, complicate the notion of "women" making informed choices about sexuality both due to the youth of the girls and their generational, economic, and/or institutional subordination to older men. Stories about young girls in relationships with or raped by older men resonate with the mgoneko stories about girls attacked in dormitories. Mgoneko stories that feature single women, particularly young women (teenagers and school girls) living in groups without men may constitute a significant variation in mgoneko tales. That is, while some mgoneko stories seem to point to women's vulnerability in marriage, stories about unmarried women living in groups may be pointing toward a different source of vulnerability or fear; they therefore call for a different interpretation from that of marital rape or domestic abuse. As I did in the previous section, I set the concerns raised in mgoneko tales about young women living in groups without men in the context of concerns raised in the media contemporaneously. One concern the media has highlighted is the role that age disparities between older men who sleep with much younger girls may play in the spread of HIV. Examining the media scrutiny surrounding such relationships helps us make sense of some variants of mgoneko tales.

In the busy trading center of Ekwendeni in 2006, girls in the dorms of a secondary school reported the horror of discovering they had been mysteriously molested in the night. Weeks later *The Nation* reported that 31 girls had been sent home from the same school suffering from strange symptoms for which doctors could find no physical cause. The girls were said to suffer from heavy shivering, failure to walk, and "mental disorder." A school administrator denied the rumors that the incident was due to a teacher practicing Satanism or witchcraft but one of the students claimed the school was trying to cover up the truth. The same young woman rejected the allegations that the afflicted girls were going home to abort pregnancies and instead asserted "One of us was actually [mysteriously] beaten [and] she was sick." While some religious leaders said Satanism could not be ruled out as a cause of the girls' ailment, Malawi's chief government psychiatrist said that the girls were likely suffering from "conversion disorder" as a result of severe stress (*The Nation*, Strange disease attacks 31 students, March 31, 2006).[5] "Conversion disorder" is what was once known as "hysteria," contagious delusions with somatic effects. The attack of girls in Ekwendeni was not the first such incident known in Malawi. Around the same time another newspaper, Malawi's *Sunday Times* reported that women in Ndirande were being haunted "by a mysterious beast since 2004." The "enigma" was said to be the work of Satanism and witchcraft. "The enigma, which only targets women, also attacked girls at Blantyre Secondary School in their hostel in April 2004 where several students were mysteriously injured" (*The Sunday Times*, Living Waters prays for tortured women February 26, 2006).

Why might teenage schools girls be perceived as endangered? Media attention given to transgenerational sex and public health campaigns pointing to dangers of early sexual debut may attribute to anxiety around teenage girls. The media has also given some attention to male teachers who sexually exploit their female students and (among other things) expose them to AIDS infection. The following articles express these concerns:

> July 19, 2001 50 teachers die every month, says minister *The Nation*
>
> Mar. 2002 1 teacher dies daily, says TUM [Teachers' Union of Malawi] *The Nation*
>
> July 19, 2005 Govt loses 6,071 teachers to HIV/AIDS related illnesses. *The Daily Times*
>
> Aug. 10, 2005 Teacher arrested for suspected rape. *The Nation*
>
> Nov. 9, 2005 AIDS heavily killing Malawian teachers. *The Daily Times*
>
> Nov. 25, 2005 Teacher gets 6 years for defiling own pupil. *The Nation*
>
> Oct. 30, 2006 Trans-generational sex worries NAC [Malawi National AIDS Commission]. *The Nation*

That young women in Ekwendeni could be sexually attacked at night and later suffer from a "mysterious" disease parallels anxieties expressed about sexual violence and AIDS. Beyond the threat arising specifically from teachers, young women are generally seen as targets of older men. In "Trans-generational sex worries NAC" an executive from the National AIDS Commission said that the organization was worried "with the prevalence of transgenerational sex where young people [women] are lured by financial returns and fall sexual prey to older partners." Drawing on statistics reported in Malawi's 2004 Demographic Health Survey (MDHS) the NAC official pointed out that HIV prevalence for women aged 15-24 was four times that of men in the same age bracket. For women aged 15 to 19 their HIV prevalence rate was nine times that of men in the same age bracket. (*The Nation*, October 30, 2006).

While sometimes young women with older men as sexual partners (and particularly married older men) are seen as predators and criticized or attacked by other women (see chapter 3: "Funny, Yet Sorrowful") mgoneko stories feature young women as manipulated victims; mgoneko stories draw attention to young women's relative powerlessness as expressed in acts of rape that take place as they lay sleeping. Indeed, concern with transgenerational sex in its most extreme form was decried in a 2005-2006 media panic emphasizing the rape of very young and even prepubescent girls and toddlers. The headlines were shocking:

Dec. 8, 2005 Man gets 8 years for defiling baby. *The Nation*

Jan. 9, 2006 Girl defiled at church gathering. *The Nation*

Jan. 14, 2006 Sharia for defilers, liars, and mutilators. *The Weekend Nation*

Jan. 24, 2006 Man in for infecting girl, 14, with HIV. *The Nation*

Feb. 10, 2006 Three convicted for raping girl, 14. *The Nation*

Feb. 24, 2006 Child abusers need stiffer punishment. *The Daily Times*

Mar. 30, 2006 Girl, 12, injured during defilement. *The Nation*

Mar. 22, 2006 Man defiles 2-year-old girl. *The Nation*

Another "Zabweka" cartoon commented on the rape of infacts (see Figure 5.3). In an editorial entitled "Of hate, gender violence," one writer commented, "If the girl-child manages to make it to school,

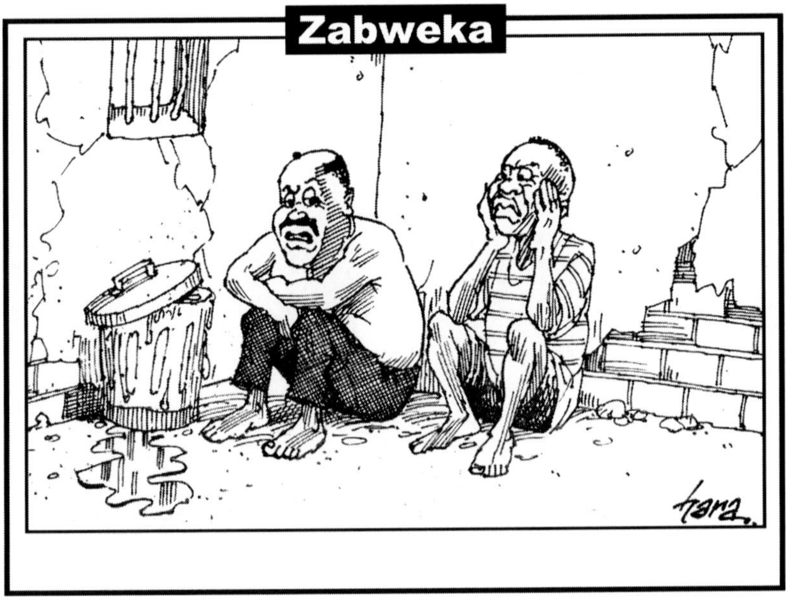

Figure 5.3 Courtesy of Nation Publications Ltd, Newspaper comic Zabweka "I'm in for molesting a two month old baby girl." By Brian Hara in *The Nation*, Dec. 15, 2005.

she is likely to face the advances of male teachers. High marks at the exams for girls are dangled as carrots to a horse in exchange for sex" (*The Nation* January 30, 2006).

However, it is not only transgenerational sex that stirs concern but also age of sexual debut. Around 2005 the American-based public health organization, Population Services International (PSI), launched a slick "multichannel intervention" campaign in select sub-Saharan African countries (Malawi, Angola, Benin, Burkina Faso, Burundi, Kenya, Togo, Zambia, Zimbabwe, Guinea, Democratic Republic of Congo) based on research linking younger ages of sexual debut with higher risks of AIDS infection. According to the DHS "Young people who initiate sex at an early age are considered to be at a higher risk of becoming pregnant or contracting an STI than young people who delay initiation of sexual activity." (NSO, 2011: 187). Through billboards, posters, and radio spots the PSI campaign urged teenagers to delay becoming sexually active until they were older.[6]

An organization that seeks to protect and promote the well-being of female students in particular is the Forum for African Women Educationalists in Malawi (FAWEMA), a nonprofit organization formed in 1993 as a branch of the Pan-African organization Forum for African Women Educationalists. FAWEMA cooperates with the government and NGOs to achieve its goal of promoting gender equity in education. FAWEMA views teenage pregnancies or sexually transmitted diseases as major barriers in girls' educations. A newspaper article entitled "Fawema keeping girls in schools" stated that in 2004, 91 boys nationally had left school due to impregnating girls while 1,834 girls has left schools due to pregnancies (*The Nation*, FAWEMA keeping girls in school, November 22, 2005). FAWEMA fought successfully to change the policy that barred girls from returning to school after pregnancy. The article went on to say that schoolboys, politicians, teachers, and other men were responsible for these pregnancies. In addition, FAWEMA is vocal in its criticism of "cultural practices" that endanger the health and well being of girls including initiation or maturity rites. In the same article FAWEMA derided the girls' maturity rites called "*chinamwali*" (or *chiputu*) saying that in some cases girls are married almost immediately after being initiated (which is usually soon after menarche). Initiation rites, the means by which gender identity and sexual mores are inculcated and kinship patterns and accompanying roles and behaviors are learned (Morris, 2000:89), may provide the imagery for mgoneko dangers to girls in dorms.

Chinamwali, female initiation rites of matrilineal peoples of central and southern Malawi, is practiced (with variation) among the Chewa, Yao, Mang'anja, as well by other peoples at the Malawi-Zambia border region. Based on the 1960s and 1970s research of van Bruegel (2001) and Brian Morris' 1990s research (2000), female novitiates are secluded as a group during the harvest season for about a week in a special hut called the *simba* (also spelled "*tsimba*") from whence they periodically go out for instructions imparted by older female initiates. "In a sense, initiations in Malawi can be viewed as a process whereby humans are gendered for the purpose of social reproduction..." (Morris, 2000: 90). Girls learn about the social and sexual aspects of womanhood by learning songs and dances as well as through various types of simulative and symbolic play. Organized by the chief, Yao *chinamwali* rites entail beer brewing, flour offerings to spirits, drawing water, and playacting. Girls are taught their responsibilities to various kin, to their husbands, and are also given instruction about sex. For example, Morris describes a ritual in which girls lie on the ground acting as if they were being attacked by ants and moving their hips to simulate sex (Morris, 2000: 90).

Perhaps most important for analysis of mgoneko dormitory attack narratives are the aspects of *chinamwali* rituals that involve the *nyau*, all-male masked secret societies. While most activities of *chinamwali* are carried out solely among girls and women, there are several points of contact between initiates and the *nyau*. These men, who dress up as various types of wild beasts, are symbolically associated with ancestral spirits, nature, and masculinity. Part of their power is in their mystery; while masked their identities are subsumed under the weight of these symbolic associations. During *chinamwali* rites the *nyau* interact with the female novitiates in ways that are sometimes playfully erotic and other times terrifying. van Bruegel described how the *nyau* (among the Chewa) would scare the girls at night:

> Late at night the girls are given some time for sleep. But even then they will not sleep much because the *Nyau* dancers come round the *tsimba*, and even push the door open, in order to frighten the girls. Even the most intrepid of girls will be scared. This enhances the idea of the mysterious character and importance of the instructions. The memory of the threatening behaviour of the *Nyau* dancers, representing the *mizimu* [spirits], will remain with them for the rest of their lives. (van Bruegel, 2001: 192)

Morris described a similar scene in which *Nyau* (among the Yao) wore claws of thorns and sprung upon girls that were reportedly misbehaving. When outside the girls' hut they banged on pots and made highly realistic sounds mimicking lion's roars and sounds of jackals (2000: 101).

Toward the end of the girls' seclusion, the *nyau* dancers engage with the women in sexually suggestive dancing:

> The masked dancers are sparsely dressed, almost naked and completely covered with old rags, grass, or banana fronds. Their heads are covered too and they wear a red headband and pieces of red cloth on their arms and legs. Approached by women, the *kasinja*[7] dance close to them, rhythmically and erotically thrusting their loins towards them. Until they are given a coin they sexually entice the women, whose gestures are not less suggestive towards the *mbalapi* [sable antelope]. (Morris, 2000: 102)

Some of the *nyau* charge the women who scatter in either fear or merriment. On the last night the *nyau* dancers appear again, called forth from the bush by the women's inviting songs. They come into the village where they dance with or chase the women and then dash back into the darkness (Morris, 2000: 105).

At the end of the last night of *chinamwali* girls who are married resume sexual relations with their husbands. Otherwise girls should sleep with their betrothed or with a designated male affine called *fisi* (hyena). Sexual intercourse is said to "warm" the girls, bringing them into adulthood. In Malawian cosmology, different stages of life (and different activities and substances) are associated with varying degrees of coldness and hotness. The very young are seen as cooler and progress into greater warmth as they age and are ushered into higher degrees of warmth through initiations. Young adults are "hot" but as one becomes an elder one cools.[8] On the last night of seclusion girls are "warmed" via sex with their husbands or a *fisi* and the rest of the community can return to regular sexual relations from which they abstained during *chinamwali*. "... [A]mong the Chewa, the unidentified man who performs this task is described as having 'eaten her maidenhood'" (Morris, 2000: 100). According to one of Morris' informants, though girls may enter the initiation lodge as virgins, they should not leave it so.

The resemblance of aspects of *chinamwali* to mgoneko in girls' dormitories is inescapable. The setting apart of girls during adolescent years for the sake of transformative learning is found in both settings. Indeed, sometimes initiations were referred to by some as "our schools," drawing an equivalence between *chinamwali* and the formal school system (Morris, 2000: 89). The frightening visitations of the *Nyau* at night are echoed by the frightful visitation of the mgoneko man. That the *Nyau* embodies both masculine and spiritual potency finds an answer in the mgoneko man who through magic rapes women. The masked and mysterious identity of *Nyau* dancers is akin to the ability of the mgoneko man to wear another face. Yet the playful and volitional aspect of interactions between novitiates and *Nyau* is missing from stories of girls who claim to be mgoneko victims. In fact, we might read mgoneko with regards to *chinamwali* initiations in two ways. First and most obviously, mgoneko stories may express fears about aspects of the initiation ceremony involving sex with a *fisi*. While long ago derided by European missionaries, rites involving *fisi* are now under attack by public health and human rights organizations as both a violation of human rights and also as risky behavior possibly spreading HIV. On a deeper level, if initiations introduce and orient a person to roles they are to play in the world and expectations of wives and lovers, then mgoneko sex is a nightmarish version of initiation in which girls are ushered into lives of violated sexuality, rape, and disease.

Initiation rituals, however, are not static institutions (what institution is?); although precolonial versions of *chinamwali* excluded the participation of male *nyau* masked dancers/wild animals, men in some uxorilocal societies increasingly gained power in matrilineages by expanding the roles of the *nyau* in ritual and social control. Kachapila asserts that by the 1920s, "Nyau enabled men to ritually subjugate women by infiltrating *chinamwali*" (Kachapila, 2006: 333). Descriptions of the *nyau* role in girls' initiations from this time involve girls being teased and beaten by *nyau* dancers. At the same time, missionaries from various denominations had begun to experiment with Christianized versions of initiations (Phiri, 1983). More recently Rachel Fiedler observed Christianized rites that included no act of sex between a male initiator and the initiates. However, it is difficult to determine whether this absence is specifically related to the Christianization of the rituals, to variation across communities, or to a general transformation taking place in Christian and non-Christian versions.

Peters, Walker, and Kambewa stated that there is no current measurement of the extent of the so-called "dangerous cultural practices" being actively engaged in at this time. However, in the context of AIDS that finds Malawians modifying both "everyday and 'cultural'" practices we may presume that these practices continue to be modified (Peters, Kambewa, and Walker, 2010: 294; cf Lwanda, 2006). Furthermore, according to Peters, secrecy around initiations may be increasing amidst the negative attention focused on them from the press, NGOs, and government (Pauline Peters, personal communications, December 2012). I am not aware of any recent ethnographic observations made of girls' initiations in Central and Southern Malawi. So while we may not have a clear idea as to the extent of the practices, the extent of the negative media attention may suffice to create a sense of danger around girls' initiations.

The media certainly plays a role in demonizing rites associated with girls' initiation and other aspects of "traditional culture." Ribohn found that after the 1994 transition to multiparty democracy, Malawian officials, pop singers, NGOs, and the media singled out several cultural practices that they labeled as violations of women's rights that encouraged domestic violence (Ribohn, 2002: 167). More than ten years after the democratic transition the refrain of abusive, dangerous, or anti-development culture has continued to be repeated. The newspaper articles whose titles are listed below tell the now familiar tale:

June 9, 2005 Ban explicit dances. *The Sunday Times*

July 12, 2005 Ngoni Chiefs Agree to Review practices. *The Nation*

July 11, 2005 Culture source of violence-CHRR [Centre for Human Rights and Rehabilitation]. *The Nation*

July 14, 2005 Men grilled at AIDS day event. *The Nation*

July 18, 2005 Gender based violence on the increase. *The Nation*

Dec. 15, 2005 Senior Chewa Chief bashes some rituals. *The Nation*

In "Senior Chewa Chief bashes some rituals," a female chief of Lilongwe complained that certain rituals were responsible for spreading HIV. She decried the practices of "widow inheritance" wherein a widowed woman marries the deceased brother/male relative, "widow cleansing" wherein a woman must sleep with a designated man to protect the family from being troubled by further deaths, and *kuchotsa fumbi* (shaking the dust) wherein "girls are forced to have sexual intercourse with men after initiation. " Senior Chief Khongoni, a woman, worried that an HIV infected *fisi* (hyena) would spread the disease to the girl and asked "[W]hat type of culture is that? We should make sure this is stopped forthwith otherwise the nation will perish..." (*The Nation*, December, 12, 2005).

Mgoneko stories set in girls' dorms are a variant of mgoneko tales that tap into fears stirred in public discourse surrounding transgenerational sex, early age of sexual debut, and "dangerous traditions." The anxiety about the future that awaits girls may partially account for these tales of sexual haunting whereby teenagers anticipate womanhood fraught with vulnerabilities vis-à-vis men. Mgoneko is the frightening initiation into that world of violated sexuality by beastly men described vividly in story after story of violent marital relationships.

Nachipanti: Hear No Evil, See No Evil

In the report "Mysterious man haunts women," a woman claimed that a mysterious man came into her locked bedroom. She called her neighbors for help and they came to pursue "it." They threw rocks but the rocks flew back at them until finally, "The phantom got angry and produced a monstrous sound that left all of us numb and it vanished into thin air." In addition, the phantom was said to have a curious habit of transferring women's underwear from one house to another. The article further asserted, "Men do not see the enigma" (*The Sunday Times*, January 2006). This is a strange assemblage of behaviors indeed! From the mysterious nature of the assailant (phantom, enigma, maker of monstrous sounds, etc.), to its visibility to women only, the mystery man captured the imaginations and stirred the fears of Malawians. The stories and commentary surrounding the mysterious man press into questions about the consequences of violence (whether aided by magic or not) and also press into questions about how authorities respond to gender-based violence.

This "phantom" became known as "*nachipanti*," meaning one wearing pants (underpants) only. He was rumored to operate in Blantyre, more specifically in the relatively impoverished section called Ndirande. The mysterious man reportedly began his activities around April 2004 by attacking girls in the Blantyre Secondary School girls dorms. The same year in May, *nachipanti* attacked a primary school teacher who sustained a brain injury from which she later died. In December 2004, two sisters living together were assaulted. One was killed while the other's injuries to the head rendered her unconscious for days. (*The Sunday Times*, "Mysterious man haunts women," January 2006). According to the informants I interviewed in Zomba in 2010, *nachipanti* entered women's homes through magic, beat them (especially on the head), raped them, and sucked their blood. One woman told me that *nachipanti* sucked women's blood through the penis and on the following day they would die from blood loss. Another informant said victims were hit on the head with a stone and then blood was drained from the head and afterwards stored in plastic bags. Informants associated *nachipanti* with Satanism and witchcraft. *Nachipanti* targeted women (especially those who were not married or lived without men) but also harmed children, could not be seen by men, and moved quickly and stealthily, entering locked homes through magic. One informant heard that through magic *nachipanti* would become a cockroach to enter through cracks. Eventually, *nachipanti* was determined to be not one person but several young men, commissioned by a female businesswoman and supported by high-level government officials to increase their wealth and influence.

Innocent Matawere, the man who apprehended Jack Bandawe (often simply referred to as "*nachipanti*" and said to be the leader of the band of thugs), said that the *nachipanti* men used magic to cause people in the vicinity of their intended victims to fall into a deep sleep so that no one would hear the victims' cries. In late 2009, Matawere was driving a female neighbor home from the hospital in the wee hours of the night when they saw a man dressed only in underpants in a yard jumping back and forth over a charcoal burner. According to Matawere, his neighbor insisted that he confront the man. He chased the man and eventually caught and beat him. Matawere said that once he had Bandawe on the ground, Bandawe tried to bribe him with money to let him go free, but Matawere rejected the bribe. When the neighbors were finally roused and gathered around the fight scene, they wanted to set *nachipanti* on fire, saying he was worse than a dog (Innocent Matawere, July 30, 2010). Meanwhile, three victims aged 17, 14 and, 3 years old were found in a house and then taken to the hospital. Bandawe was taken to the police where he identified his accomplices. He was later put on trial and sentenced to death.

Nachipanti stories combine elements from several dramatic and/or gory genres. Bloodsucking tales, known throughout central Africa, have been circulating for almost a century (see Luise White (2000)). Mgoneko motifs are incorporated, as are the sensational elements of media stories about physically abused women and girls. In *nachipanti*, you find mgoneko magic, house breaking, theft, beating, blood sucking, rape, community or authoritative responses, and government conspiracy. Here, I focus on two motifs of *nachipanti* stories: the invisibility of *nachipanti* to men and the ability of *nachipanti* to make neighbors deaf to the cries of victims. Both of these motifs express concerns about the failure of people to intervene or take responsibility of acknowledging and punishing gender-based abuses.

Nachipanti stories may be thought of as extreme mgoneko tales owing to their greater level of violence and the heightened fear surrounding *nachipanti*. As with other mgoneko stories, *nachipanti*'s violence is possible because of the ability of the perpetrator to put people into a deep sleep through magic. Unlike other mgoneko stories, it is not merely the victim herself who is put to sleep but the people living around her. In other words, for violence to go on people in the community have to be oblivious to it, to not hear screams. These features of *nachipanti* pose a curious contrast to motifs in stories told about women who felt silenced in the colonial regimes of Central Africa (White, 2000: 117-121). Instead of women being silenced, in *nachipanti* stories women struggle and scream but are not heard. Some people in the community are more oblivious to *nachipanti* than others. *Nachipanti* were not visible to men, making men both blind and deaf to the violence perpetuated by the beast/phantom/enigma.

The idea that women are speaking up and not being heard brings up questions of collective responsibility, authority, and accountability. Whose responsibility is it to respond to and bring an end to violence against women and girls? Who has been responsible thus far and who has failed to respond? According to Matawere's account, he was at first reluctant to intervene when he saw Jack Bandawe in the yard. He told himself that perhaps the strange man wearing only underpants and jumping about belonged where he was, that the man was the husband of the woman within the house, that the couple had a strange relationship. In other words, what was going on was private, none of his business. It was at the urging of his female friend, that he intervened. Though he could physically see the *nachipanti* man and what he was doing, he could not see that he was a problem until a woman insisted that what he was seeing was problematic. Only then did he react.

After turning over Jack Bandawe to police Matawere claims that police and other government authorities were hiding the truth of what was really happening with *nachipanti*, his accomplices, and their boss. The theme of crimes not taken seriously by authorities is one echoed in other stories circulating about cases of rape and gender-based violence. Several journalers I worked with reported stories about rapes that contained explicit criticism of village heads, police, Traditional Authorities (chiefs over lower level villages heads with official government status as keepers of the peace and assistants to District Commissioners), and elder relatives. While *nachipanti* Jack Bandawe was sentenced to life imprisonment for one count of attempted murder and sentenced to death for two counts of murder, other alleged rapists are not punished. Journaler Simon Nyirenda reported a story told to him by a middle-aged man named Mr. Mpaso. Mpaso gossiped about a man named Mr. Nyasulu who was reputed to be a brutal wife beater. According to Mpaso, the man had even been seen beating his wife in public. In late 2008, Nyasulu was accused of raping a young schoolgirl (age 14) as she walked home from class. After the rape, the girl shouted for help "but it was already too late and Nyasulu had vanished." The girl told her uncle (who was her caretaker and guardian) and he brought her to confront Nyasulu that same night. Nyasulu did not admit guilt, so the uncle and the girl went to the village headman who advised them to report the matter to the police:

> Mpaso: But alas! The same night we heard that Mr Nyasulu sent two of his workers to the uncle of the girl with a K 20 000 to seal up his mouth. In fact the money which was given to him was actually meant to make the uncle of the girl to drop the matter. The uncle received the money and he really called off the case. He did not even go to the police station to report the matter. The following morning the people were just wondering to see that the man was no longer looking to be interested with the matter. After investigations they actually found out that the uncle of the girl had been given money by Nyasulu. Then the matter ended up just like that, so you can imagine that what kind of a person is he [Nyasulu]? He is better off because he has money which helps him to be able to put down the serious cases that he normally provokes. (Simon Nyirenda research journal. Rumphi, September/ Octotober 2008)

In this case, the storyteller feels that the victim's uncle failed in his responsibility of pursuing a criminal case against Nyasulu. Mpaso, who related this story to the journaler went on to say that the story of this young girl was similar to those he had heard on the radio. On the radio he heard of a young girl being raped and infected with HIV. He suspected that the girl raped by Mr. Nyasulu was probably infected with HIV as well. Rape has become equated with murder by way of HIV.

In a case reported by another journaler, Hastings Mkandawire, a village head (50 years old) stood accused of raping a young girl (15 years old). While Mkandawire was getting his bike repaired at the bike repair shop, people standing around spoke about the scandalous case. It was said that the headman was not going to be punished because the case was being handled by the Traditional Authority who was a friend of the accused. Those in the conversation scoffed at the accused's defense that he had an agreement with the girl wherein he gave her money and she gave him sex. Someone said that the man was unscrupulous because he used his relative privilege to avoid punishment for his crime:

> "Only that Jalasi [the alleged rapist] took an advantage that the parents of the girl are poor and not educated. Had it been the parents were educated enough they would have taken him to police as a sexual abuse/rape [case]. The girl is about 15 years old and takes him a man about 50 years old?" (Hastings Mkandawire research journal, Rumphi, October 22, 2008)

In a case reported by another journaler Tawonga Msowoya, a man was caught trying to rape his own mother. The mother woke up and screamed and neighbors came to rescue her and catch the culprit.[9] The man fled the scene and it took a week to track him down. The woman relating the events said that the case was in the hands of the police and would go to the court soon. The journaler responded by saying that it was good that the case was being handled by the government courts because the chief would have probably taken a bribe. The opinion of people telling these stories is that prosecuting rape cases is the responsibility of government courts rather than traditional authorities (Tawonga Msowoya research journal, Rumphi, January 26, 2006). These narratives shared in villages form a part of a broader national discourse aired in newspapers that not only calls for traditional authorities such as chiefs and village heads to productively intervene in gender-based violence, but also call for the government to intensify its response to rape and molestation.

Malawi's news media produced numerous articles and opinion pieces questioning what was being done by authorities to curb and punish rape and what should be done. Of these articles, the following serve as a sample:

Dec. 14, 2005 051214 "Deal with rapists." *The Nation*

Jan. 12, 2006 060112 "Chief in on rape charge." *The Nation*

Jan. 14, 2006 060114 "Sharia for defilers, liars, and mutilators." *The Weekend Nation*

Jan. 18, 2006 060118 "On molestation, wife battering." *The Nation*

Jan. 24, 2006 060124 "Govt proposes bill to curb domestic violence." *The Nation*

Jan. 30, 2006 060130 "Of hate, gender violence." *The Nation*

Feb. 24, 2006 060224 "Child abusers deserve stiffer punishment." *The Daily Times*

Feb. 24, 2006 060224 "This Abuse needs a new approach." *The Daily Times*

Mar. 24, 2006 060324 "Resident magistrates to handle rape cases." *The Nation*

Mar. 13, 2006 "Govt urges chiefs to curb violence." *The Nation*

One common suggestion made was for a broad-based response, a commenter wrote:

> Time has come for everybody who can do something to act. It is high time society broke this silence upheld by tradition of non-interference into other people's family affairs. NGOs should be more pro-active in their interventions. They should not wait for these barbarious [sic] acts to happen and then only come in to condemn them. Above all else, we expect the law enforcers to move with speed in investigating such matters and the law to take its course against offenders. (*The Nation*, "Increased cases of violence sickening," January 24, 2006)

Another commenter in an opinion piece published a month later also called for a "multisectoral" approach whereby NGOs along with religious, political, and traditional leaders should play a role in eliminating sexual offenses. More specifically he called for a proactive approach of sensitizing people in rural areas to their rights in order to "nip the evil in the bud before it comes out to haunt women and innocent children." (*The Daily Times*, "This Abuse need a new approach," February 24, 2006).

Taken together such public and informal discourse spreads the blame around, sometimes calling for specific groups of people or authorities to take greater responsibility in enforcing women rights. Men, the government, and traditional leaders (village heads and chiefs) are urged to take greater responsibility for safe guarding women and leading the rural masses to improved women's rights. This discourse has consequences. The persistent criticism of government lenience in sentencing rapists resulted in a change in the way rape cases are handled. In March 2006, Chief Justice Leonard Unyolo decreed that rape and defilement cases had to be handled in upper courts rather in lower courts. While lower court magistrates were constrained to handing down prison sentences of a maximum 5 years, Chief Resident Magistrates (of which there are only four in Malawi) can hand down sentences of up to 14 years. A court official confirmed that the change was made as a result of "complaints by the public that convicted rapists and defilers are given lenient sentences." (*The Nation*, "Resident magistrates to handle rape cases," February. 24, 2006)

When read as part of a media panic over sexual assaults, the *nachipanti* stories express some of the frustrations involved in pursuing justice in a rape case. In particular, the failure of men to recognize and acknowledge acts of rape is featured as blindness. With regard to the *nachipanti*, some thought that the case would not be fully pursued by the criminal justice system. Similar concerns are echoed in research journal reports about rape cases lacking national notoriety. A repeated theme therein was one of the unreliability of traditional local authorities as arbiters of rape cases. Some people saw chiefs and headman and male elders as susceptible to bribes and prone to set aside their responsibility to victims by not pursuing punishment beyond a fine. By contrast, rape was seen as a problem that is within the jurisdiction of government police rather than local or familial authorities.

These stories may also portray confusion over the process of seeking justice. A woman's path to reporting a civil or criminal complaint has been documented by the Women and Law in Southern Africa Research and Educational Trust (WLSA). The 2000 WLSA report on women's access to justice found that depending on the nature of the crime and their relationship to the perpetrator, women sought justice for assault and rape by approaching chiefs, NGOs, district commissioners, churches, marriage counselors, and the police. WLSA described the processes through which women proceeded as a maze, perplexing and not straightforward and especially difficult in rural areas (WLSA, 2000: 23). While the experience of seeking justice may be confusing, *nachipanti* and mgoneko stories make the case that all men and multiple institutions ought to bear responsibility for intervening in cases of gender-based violence. The popularity of mgoneko stories suggest that some aspects of the message of women's rights and some general knowledge of legal reforms spread by NGOS, governmental agencies, and the media have extended into the rural areas even while the infrastructure for dispensing justice for women has not been fully constructed. For example, in a village in Mchinji I was told by my informants that they had heard about the Victims Support Unit, a police division specially trained to deal with issues relating to abuse of women and children. The village head had begged the group to come and sensitize the people of his village, but they had never shown up. He wanted the police to explain things about women's rights because he believed villagers would take the issues more seriously if informed by police rather than by the chief (Victor Ziwa, Mchinji, July 26, 2010). *Nachipanti* stories remind us of how easy it is for a rapist to slip away and vanish even while people are desperately calling for help.

Discussion

Mgoneko stories constitute a discourse about rape and responsibility. These narratives, though portraying the fantastic, magical, and gruesome, also portray the mundane, the way in which sexual abuse is routine, culturally embedded, invisible, or unacknowledged and unpunished. The popularity of these stories in various forms and disseminated via various media attest to the regrettable plausibility of the tales to those who share them and listen to them. What makes rumor, gossip, and contemporary legend compelling is that they are propositions of truth about the world. The world as conjured and portrayed in *nachipanti* stories is a world in which a community can be deaf to the cries of people in need and a world where men are blind to abuse against women. Mgoneko stories about young women in dorms are akin to violent sexual initiations, precursors for a life of disempowerment in the bedroom. And mgoneko stories in which women are attacked in their own bedrooms (sometimes when husbands are near) express the sense that the home is not necessarily a haven from harm. The mass media milieu in which these stories take shape provides a vital reference point for interpreting mgoneko stories. The media may have indeed helped to stir a panic around the issue of gender-based violence and in this way they may count themselves successful. However, this success in "sensitizing" the public may have yielded some unintended consequences.

Because mgoneko stories involve magic some may be tempted to see them as metaphor or fantasy. But mgoneko stories not only have metaphorical significance but some may arise from experiences and give rise to material consequences. Mgoneko stories may be associated with differing types of experiences from sleep paralysis to erotic dreams to physical rape. The fear created by a mgoneko experience or by being told that one has unknowingly been subject to a mgoneko attack has lead some women to go for HIV testing, others to consult traditional healers, and lead some communities to fine, expel, or report suspected culprits to the government police. Indeed, in a case believed to involve mgoneko magic Jack Bandawe, *nachipanti*, was arrested and convicted of murder. Folklorists who study contemporary legend call the relationship between narrative and action "ostension" (Goldstein, 2004: 29). Mgoneko stories, told as plausible and possibly, deal in real life conflicts and produce real life consequences in some instances.

The media panic surrounding gender-based violence may have helped to stir narrative ostension around mgoneko and fuel fears about women's vulnerability. The attention that media gave to not only the details of gruesome assaults, but also their portrayal of increasingly prevalent violence against women and young girls, and possible links between HIV infection and rape, explain the alarm some felt when hearing about mgoneko stories. These tales that weave together reports circulated in the national press with rumors of events on the local level, are a plea for greater intervention, they relate the confusion of who is officially responsible for punishing gender-based violence, they expose the shame of authorities failing in their responsibility, and they suggest there are places that human rights and more specifically women's rights have not reached.

CONCLUSION

In this book I have shown how rumor, gossip, advice, and legend surrounding marriage- and sex-related conflicts in a time of AIDS serve as powerful means by which people (especially wives here) both express and mitigate their sense of vulnerability. While Western media, various nongovernmental organizations, and numerous scholars have pointed out the vulnerability of women in countries of Africa where AIDS is endemic, I have sought not to deny women's vulnerability, but to portray it in the popular imagery of Malawians. In doing so I have found that narratives serve as powerful sources of critique, following the tradition of women's pounding songs and possession cults. While women's spiritual possession served as critique of growing male political and economic dominance in the colonial era, possession and the healing practices that evoked possession were also meant to be a means by which society was transformed. Similarly, the knowledge and advice women gather is meant to be "good medicine," providing a balm to heal relationships, rather than reject marriage (as an institution), their husbands, and the family obligations and privileges entailed in marriage. These relationships are both a strength and hardship. Women who harness the power of gossip among relatives and neighbors to oust a romantic rival, for example, may find themselves in a similar position in that same milieu at a later date. Marriage, while holding out the promise of greater relational and financial stability for a couple, is fraught with difficult decisions that cause strains in relationships. Stories about the use of love potions and travel charms reveal the tensions engendered by male labor migration. Indeed, labor migration (especially long distance) and happy marriage and family life are seen as opposed in some of these tales. No good solution is posited to resolve these tensions but rather stories of love potions and witch baskets, as well as those about fighting rivals, reveal the need for people to make constant trade-offs and negotiations. These stories reject easy answers to complex problems.

On a larger scale, fears of hidden abuses in male–female sexual relationships or hidden disease status are portrayed in *mphutsi* and *mgoneko* rumors. These stories tell us that as the AIDS epidemic has matured in Malawi, old anxieties about who is at risk for sexually transmitted disease reemerges, revealing that beliefs about guilty disease transmitters in the form of prostitutes and male migrant laborers have never been completely submerged by the generalized epidemic. At the same time, the desire for clear categories of who is diseased and therefore guilty and who is well and therefore innocent show a kind of nostalgia for the early days of the AIDS epidemic when "at risk" groups were primarily targeted for interventions. With the growth of the generalized epidemic and the recent proliferation of drugs that can (to some extent) help mask HIV serostatus, AIDS is now both less threatening and more difficult to detect at the same time. With *mgoneko* stories, concerns about the hidden abuses in relationships are brought to light. The conjunction of media attention brought to bear on spousal abuse, teachers' molestation of female students, and certain initiation rites serves as the context for the emergence of scares over *mgoneko* magic. These stories are a barely disguised call for various authorities as well as men in general to pay attention and take responsibility for gender-based violence. Some *mgoneko* stories speak of women who are attacked in the night by magical seducers/rapists while their husbands lie asleep and unable to help them. Furthermore, tales of the *nachipanti* killer of Ndirande, Blantyre describe a violent culprit who was not visible to men, but attacked women only in the dead of night. *Mgoneko* stories enjoin men to open their ears and awaken to the abuse of women that is taking place in their communities and maybe even in their own marriages.

I began my project by pursuing questions about narratives that circulated in familial circles, among friends, relatives, and neighbors. But as I was completing it I saw that some narratives were making their rounds in wider fields, such as in the news media. While gossip has the potential to impact individuals in a tight knit community, rumors circulating more broadly have the potential to make over societies and shift attitudes, attention, and even laws, as noted in chapter 5. The content of the narrative matters, but the forums through which stories circulate also matter. This insight is leading me into a new direction of inquiry. Spaces where stories are powerfully deployed are in legal forums. Malawi is in the midst of sweeping legislative reform of laws to protect women and enhance their status in society. In 2008 and 2010, I collected hundreds of District court transcripts of marital dispute cases.

These narratives are not merely a record of how enacted laws are enforced, they also express ways that people catch hold of changing national rhetoric around gender and human rights to shape it to their own ends. Interviews I conducted in 2010 suggest that women's rights laws have opened up a new space for women to negotiate their rights in everyday life as district courts and police have in the last few years made greater efforts to protect women from various forms of abuse and disempowerment. The passage of the 2006 Prevention of Domestic Violence Act is one major catalyst. Therein the idea of "abuse" has been considerably expanded to include not only physical abuse but also economic and emotional abuse. Yet a man I interviewed (a village head) was eager to express his concern that gender rights had gone too far. He wondered, "Who would protect us men from women?" Other headmen, trained in implementing women's rights law were willing to implement some aspects of the law, but were wary of "foreign" or offensive notions such as the idea of marital rape saying explicitly that the laws needed to be sensitive to local culture. Meanwhile, two women saw gender rights embodied in the activities of the Community Police, volunteer lay police trained by government police agencies. Their neighbor and friend often suffered violence at the hands of her husband. She had recently been given a bell to ring to alert the Community Police. On one occasion the Community Police responded by tying up the culprit and pouring onto him a plant substance that made him itch in agony all night long.

At the same time, an overwhelming majority of divorce cases tried in district courts are brought by disgruntled wives. Many women call upon evolving notions of rights and responsibilities to make their cases in vivid narratives of abuse, neglect, and alienation of affection. Yet some village elders complain that now there are too many divorces and too many women bypassing the authority of elders and village councils to negotiate marital conflicts. Other elders actively engage in court processes, supporting their daughters and sisters. My preliminary research suggests that women are finding these government courts a powerful venue for revealing secrets and shaping narratives in ways that can reshape their lives.

NOTES

1 Introduction

1. The Malawi Diffusion and Ideational Change Project has been funded by the National Institute of Child Health and Human Development (NICHD), grants R01–37276, R01-HD44228–01, R01-HD050142, R01-HD/MH-41713–0. The MDICP has also been funded by the Rockefeller Foundation, grant RF-99009#199. The MDICP received ethical approval from institutional review boards at the University of Pennsylvania and the University of Malawi.
2. We used NVivo software for coding the ethnographic journals.
3. Catherine was pregnant with her first child when we began conducting interviews at the end of 2005.
4. The approach was developed by or associated with Mitchell (1956); Turner (1996[1957]); Epstein (1958); van Velsen (1964); Marwick (1965); Long (1968); Kapferer (1972).
5. The names of journalers as well as the names of the people to whom they refer are anonymized. The journalers' editorial comments are italicized and placed in parentheses. I have edited rumor journal quotes for readability. All changes are made with the intention of maintaining the rhythm and imagery of the original report. Most of my "corrections" are simply breaking up and punctuating run-on sentences. My additions of missing words are in square brackets. Other corrections include correcting spellings, adjusting subject-verb agreement, and adding articles. I have avoided inverting sentence syntax and other substantive changes.
6. By "relevant conversation" I refer to discussions that are pertinent to this particular research agenda.
7. "chiTumbuka" means the language of the Tumbuka. The prefix "chi" means "language of."
8. Two journalers lived within the same village, two lived in Rumphi township, and another journaler lived half a mile outside the township.
9. The village name is a pseudonym to protect the identity of my informants.

10. Convenience store for the sale of manufactured consumer goods such as soaps, razors, packaged snack food, and other consumable convenience items.
11. Smearing refers to resurfacing both the exterior and interior of the hut with mud, which is used as plaster.
12. *Chichewa* meaning getting thinner and thinner.
13. For a discussion of advice, see also Swidler and Watkins (2005). "Hearsay Ethnography."
14. Gary Alan Fine mentions that advice is one function of contemporary legends (also known as urban legends), as contemporary legends "are designed to be spread to relevant others who care and who might face similar situations" (1992:30).

2 Advice Is Good Medicine: Marriage, Advice, and The Comforts of Home

1. Though widely practiced, polygamy rates vary across marriage types (e.g., it is more prevalent in patrilineal unions than martrilineal). However, polygamy is not the only type of "multiple and concurrent sexual partnerships" (MCP) practiced in Malawi. Chirwa and Chizimbi's report identifies numerous types of MCP men and women engage in though polygamy was an option open exclusively to men (2009). Chirwa and Chizimbi's informants, interviewed in focus groups, were asked to distinguish between polygamy and infidelity/extramarital affairs. According to some of the men interviewed extramarital affairs was generally described as taking place secretly such that a man's wife was not told directly about the affair. With an affair, as opposed to a courtship for marriage, the "other" woman was not sanctioned by the relatives of the man as a potential wife, nor were "proper procedures" for marital incorporation as with a polygamous courtship and union. Interviewees said a girlfriend in an affair with a married man does not have recognized claim on the man's property as a wife does. Some of the women interviewed saw little difference between polygamous unions and extramarital affairs, some claiming that girlfriends can benefit from even greater material support than a wife. Some of the adolescent girls said as much adding that "it is a practice that violates our rights" (Chirwa and Chizimbi, 2009: 30–31).
2. For more on the development of prevention strategies in Malawi, see Baylies and Bujra (2000); Poulin (2007); and Watkins (2004).
3. Bridewealth among the Tumbuka is usually paid in cattle and/or cash.
4. This proverb seems to be a combination of two or more Biblical references. The first is "There is nothing new under the sun," which

is found in Ecclesiastes 1:8. The second part of the proverb more specifically speaks of the revelation of secrets with reference to the light metaphor found in the New Testament. See, for example, 1 Corinthians 3:13. "[H]is work will be shown for what it is, because the Day will bring it to light." (Bible, New International Version)

5. "Proposing" a woman does not mean proposing marriage but is a common expression for a man proposing a romantic, sexual relationship to a woman.
6. Schatz has also noted in her qualitative research conducted in rural Malawi (including Rumphi District) that respondents claimed that reports of infidelity always required further proving (2002: 309).
7. Talking "anyhow" means to express your anger freely or to speak without thought and consideration to consequences.
8. Schmidt found similar experiences among nineteenth century Shona women who called themselves strangers and referred to their in-laws as "owners." (1992: 17). Lloyd (1968) talks about the "stranger" status of young Yoruba wives in their virilocalities. Richards, in a study conducted in the early decades of the twentieth century, found that the matrilocal Chewa of what is now central Malawi "talk of the father as a stranger." (Richards, 1950: 233)
9. When a woman refuses to "eat," what she is really doing is refusing to be eaten. The folktale variant in which the husband is a python who visits his wife at night under the cover of darkness and partially swallows her makes the link between eating and sexual intercourse explicit (Bill, 1994: 58–59). Linguistically the distinction is even built into the words "to marry," which vary according to gender. Among the Tumbuka, men take a wife (*kutenga*) while women are taken (*kutengwa*). (Turner, 1996 [1952]).
10. Phukwa is a marketplace close to the village. The market or the town is associated with youth, uncontrolled sexuality, and AIDS. For a discussion of the perceived link between youth, mobility, commodities, sexuality, and AIDS, cf. Setel (1999).
11. A similar complaint is made by women in South Africa. Informants of Harrison and Montgomery talked about the problems of men changing after the wedding and complained about difficulties of living with in-laws. "'It's difficult at other people's houses. God gives you strength to be patient, but you often think about leaving. Men will treat you well for the first few months. He'll change after 6–7 months. It's difficult! I don't even know how much he earns [now]." (Harrison and Montgomery, 2001: 317).
12. Gogo means grandparent. "A" is a prefix used as an honorific or when directly addressing an individual.
13. Our informant seemed to believe that the husband in her story was bringing his first wife to meet the new wife out of cruelty rather than

out of a practical motive. Husbands may want to make sure cowives can get along, and thus an introduction would be a matter of practicality. Here, however, the narrator was intent upon creating an image of a mean husband.

14. Ruth Chirwa's extraordinary story will be explored further in the next chapter.
15. "Cooking" and "food," particularly *nyama*, which is beef or flesh; *nsima,* which is maize porridge and the staple food; or *maswiti,* which are candies, are associated with sex.
16. Janet Bujra also reports similar complaints heard among elders in Tanzania. The sense that youth fail to listen was supported by AIDS literature in Tanzania, which in early days focused heavily on youth (2000).
17. Indeed, Estery's own husband began an extramarital relationship when they moved to the city of Lilongwe. When he refused to end the relationship, she grew fearful of contracting AIDS, so she went back to their village to raise their children and left him with the other woman. He visited her once and tried to initiate sex and she refused him. He returned to the city to stay with his other woman. When he became ill, he returned to the area to be treated at the Livingstonia hospital where Estery visited to take care of him. The health personnel at the hospital told her he was dying of AIDS.
18. Malawians often translate the term *ndiwo* as "relish," but the better English equivalent might be "side dish."

3 Funny, Yet Sorrowful: Narratives of Empowerment and Empathy in Woman Against Woman Struggles

1. Journalers were instructed to give dialogue-style accounts of conversations in which information relating to sex, AIDS, and religion was discussed rather than simply summarize conversations. However, sometimes journalers would write summaries such as the one included here. This was especially the case for new journalers. In Chipeta's excerpt, he has summarized information from several conversations that took place in his village.
2. A kind of machete used locally usually for agricultural purposes and sometimes for butchering meat.
3. Veranda or stoop.
4. Of first marriages 40 percent of respondents in the MDICP Rumphi sample were polygamous in 2001. Sixty-five percent of second marriages were polygamous. (Reniers, 2003: 188).
5. AIDS prevention campaigns carried out by government and NGOs in Malawi often describe their educational tasks as "sensitizing" the masses.

4 "Nobody Fears AIDS, *MPHUTSI* is More Fire": Disease Rumors in the Age of AIDS Treatment

1. In Malawi, the belief that innocent people can suffer sickness because of the wrongdoings of others is a part of the Malawian conceptions of disease pre-dating the advent of AIDS. According to Morris, literature on African disease concepts have identified four broad categories of disease causation, which are also evident among the Chewa of Southern Malawi: natural diseases or those "from God," those deriving from moral infringement, afflictions caused by witchcraft or sorcery (*matsenga*, that is, magic), and spirit-induced afflictions (Brian Morris and Peters et al.). Illnesses caused by a violation of some ritual or moral interdiction are said to cause suffering to those connected to the violators. A few examples of such diseases include tsempho, likango, and ndaka (Morris, 1996: 130). In particular, ideas about the cause of tsempho (also called mdulo) seem to bear a strong resemblance to ideas expressed about both AIDS and mphutsi. Morris describes the disease as follows: "It is considered to be a particular kind of wasting disease that may have fatal consequences if counter-measures are not taken in the form of medicines. The disease is related to promiscuous sexual relationships, or to indulging in sexual intercourse by spouses during ritually prohibited periods. The disease affects men, women, and young children, and is caused by another's transgression." (Morris, 1996: 132)
2. In chapter 3 where I write about women who seek to separate their husbands' from extramarital partners I make a similar observation. Although some women try to label others as morally and physically sick and thus a danger to the community, it is difficult to make these stigmatizing labels stick especially as people can easily picture themselves in the same problems as the potentially stigmatized individual.

5 *MGONEKO*: Magical Rape, Media Panic, and Gender-Based Violence

1. Shevory suggests that his mass media focused usage of moral panic/media panic is closer to Cohen's original meaning than the usage of other scholars who have extended to term to study panics that occurred before the age of widely available newspapers and radio and television broadcasting.
2. Author's emphasis.
3. Accessed online June 26, 2012 at http://news.bbc.co.uk/2/hi/africa/1728875.stm.

4. Indeed, some of the women we interviewed said that people in the community did not take further direct action against the alleged mgoneko men because of the "tight security" of police who protected the mgoneko man and seized the accusing diviner.
5. The bracketed words in this quotation were inserted by the newspaper article's author, Edwin Nyirongo.
6. In Malawi, about 14 percent of women aged 15–24 said they had initiated sexual activity before age 15. By contrast, about 22 percent of men in the same age group had initiated sexual activity by age 15 (NSO, 2011: 187).
7. *Nyau* character type associated with abandoned field and represents the wild, sexual, and the untamed (Morris, 2000: 102).
8. Sexual intercourse and blood (menstrual blood in particular) are associated with being "hot" but are seen as incommensurate with periods where coldness predominates such as after a death or when a child is born. These times call for abstinence, sometimes for the individual couple, sometimes for a community as a whole. During the period in which *chinamwali* rites are taking place, not only must the novitiates abstain from sex but also the rest of the community must abstain as well (van Breugel, 2001:169–209).
9. According to the journaler, people in the community said that the man was raping his mother on advice from a traditional healer who had told him to activate the medicine for gaining riches he needed to sleep with his mother. Other explanations for suggested by commenters of rape in defilement stories was that the accused were under the influence of alcohol or marijuana or that they slept with young girls as a way to be cured of HIV infection.

REFERENCES

Abrahams, Roger. 1970. A performance-centered approach to gossip. *Man, New Series* 5(Jun.): 290–301.

Amaro, Hortensia. 1995. Love, sex, and power: considering women's realities in HIV prevention. *American Psychologist* 50(Jun.): 437–447.

Ashforth, Adam. 1996. Of secrecy and the commonplace: witchcraft and power in Soweto. *Social Research* 64(3): 1183–1234.

Ashforth, Adam. 2002. An epidemic of witchcraft? The implications of AIDS for the post-apartheid state *African Studies* 61(1): 121–142.

Ashforth, Adam. 2005. *Witchcraft, violence, and democracy in South Africa.* Chicago: University of Chicago Press.

Auslander, Mark. 1993. "Open the wombs!": The symbolic politics of modern Ngoni witchfinding. In *Modernity and its Malcontents: Ritual Power in Postcolonial Africa*, ed. Jean Comaroff and John Comaroff. 167–192. Chicago: University of Chicago Press.

Bahre, Erik. 2002. Witchcraft and the exchange of sex, blood, and money among Africans in Cape Town, South Africa. *Journal of Religion in Africa* 32(3): 300–334.

Barnard, Frans. 2005. The virgin cleansing myth: a threat to human security? Master's thesis, Royal Roads University.

Barnes, John A. 1951. *Marriage in a Changing Society: a study in structural change among the Fort Jameson Ngoni.* Rhodes-Livingstone Papers, 21. Capetown: Oxford University Press.

Barthes, Roland. 1972. *Mythologies.* New York: Hill and Wang.

Baylies, Carolyn and Janet Bujra, eds. 2000. *AIDS, sexuality and gender in Africa: Collective strategies and struggles in Tanzania and Zambia.* London: Routledge.

Becker, Howard. 1963. *Outsiders: studies in the sociology of deviance.* New York: Free Press.

Bill, Mary. 1994. Refusal to eat and drink: a metaphor for 'safe sex' in Tsonga folktales. *African Languages and Cultures* 7(1): 49–77.

Bird, Elizabeth. 1996. C.J.'s revenge: media, folklore, and the cultural construction of AIDS. *Critical Studies in Mass Communication* 13: 44–58.

Blake, Fred. 1978. Death and abuse in marriage laments: the curse of Chinese brides. *Asian Folklore Studies* 37(1): 13–33.

Booth, Karen. 2004. *Local women, global science: fighting AIDS in Kenya*. Bloomington, IN: Indiana University Press.

Boyd, Raymond and Richard Fardon. 1998. Saved by a song: patriarchy and women's experience in Chamba tellings of "The girl who wanted an unblemished husband." *Journal of African Cultural Studies* 11(Jun.): 5–25.

Brunvand, Jan H. 1981. *The vanishing hitchhiker: American urban legends and their meanings*. New York: W. W. Norton and Company.

Bujra, Janet. 2000. Target practice: gender and generational struggles in AIDS prevention work in Lushoto. In *AIDS, Sexuality and Sender in Africa: Collective Strategies and Struggles in Tanzania and Zambia*, ed. Carolyn Baylies and Janet Bujra. 114–142. London: Routledge.

Burke, Carol. 1989. Marching to Vietnam. *The Journal of American Folklore* 102(406): 424–441.

Caldwell, John, et al. 1997. Perceived male sexual needs and male sexual behaviour in Southwest Nigeria. *Social Science & Medicine* 44(8): 1195–1207.

Campbell, Catherine. 2003. *'Letting them die': why HIV/AIDS prevention programmes fail*. Bloomington and Indianapolis: Indiana University Press.

Chanock, Martin. 1998. *Law, custom and social order: the colonial experience in Malawi and Zambia*. Portsmouth, NH: Heinemann.

Chimbiri, Agnes 2007. The condom is an intruder in marriage: evidence from rural Malawi. *Social Science and Medicine* 64(5): 1102–1115.

Chimwaza, Agnes and Susan Cotts Watkins. 2004. Giving care to people with symptoms of AIDS in rural sub-Saharan Africa. *AIDS Care* Oct 16(7): 795–807.

Chirambo, Reuben. 2002. "Mzimu wa soldier": contemporary popular music and politics in Malawi. In *A Democracy of Chameleons: Politics and Culture in the New Malawi*. ed. Harri Englund. 103–122. Blantyre: CLAIM/MABUKU.

Chirwa, Wiseman. 1997. "No TEBA... Forget TEBA": the plight of Malawian ex-migrant workers to South Africa, 1988–1994. *International Migration Review* 31(3): 628–654.

Chirwa, Wiseman and Steven Chizimbi. 2009. Multiple and concurrent sexual partnerships in Malawi: a formative qualitative study. Prepared for Research to Prevention by the Summit Consulting Group.

Clark, Shelley. 2005. Perceptions of HIV risks among couples in Malawi: why do wives worry more? Presented at the Annual Meeting of the Population Association of America, April.

Clark, Shelley, et al. 2009. Marital aspirations, sexual behaviors, and HIV /AIDS in rural Malawi. *Journal of Marriage and Family* 71(May): 396–416.

Cohen, Stanley. 1972. Folk devils and moral panics: the creation of mods and rockers. London: MacGibbon and Kee Ltd.

Comaroff, Jean and John Comaroff. 1993. Introduction. In *Modernity and Its Malcontents: Ritual Power in Postcolonial Africa*, ed. by Jean Comaroff and John Comaroff. xi–xxxvii. Chicago: University of Chicago Press.

Craddock, Susan. 2000. Disease, social identity, and risk: rethinking the geography of AIDS. *Transactions of the Institute of British Geographers, New Series* 25(2): 153–168.

Dahlitz, M. and Parkes, J. D. 1993. Sleep Paralysis. *Lancet* 341 (8842): 406.

Deluz, Ariane. 1987. Social and symbolic values of feminine *Kne* initiation among the Guro of the Ivory Coast. *Transformations of African Marriage*, eds. David Parkin and David Nyamwaya. 113–135. Manchester: Manchester University Press.

Department of Nutrition, HIV and AIDS [Government of Malawi]. 2005. Malawi HIV and AIDS monitoring and evaluation report 2005. December 2005.

Department of Nutrition, HIV and AIDS [Government of Malawi] 2010–11. 2012. Global AIDS response progress report: Malawi Country report for 2010 and 2011.

Douglas, Mary. 1966. *Purity and danger: an analysis of concepts of pollution and taboo*. New York: Praeger.

Douglas, Mary. 1991. Witchcraft and leprosy: two strategies of exclusion. *Man, New Series* 26(4): 723–736.

Doyal, Lesley. 1995. *What makes women sick: gender and the political economy of health*. New Brunswick. NJ: Rutgers University Press.

Dundes, Alan and Thomas Hauschild. 1983. Auschwitz jokes. *Western Folklore* 42(4): 249–260.

Englund, Harri. 2002a. *From war to peace on the Mozambique-Malawi borderlands*. Edinburgh: Edinburgh University Press Ltd.

Englund, Harri. 2002b. Introduction: the culture of chameleon politics. In *A Democracy of Chameleons: Politics and culture in the new Malawi*. ed. Harri Englund. 11–24. Blantyre: CLAIM/MABUKU.

Englund, Harri. 2006. *Prisoners of freedom: human rights and the African poor*. Berkeley: University of California Press.

Epstein, A. L. 1958. *Politics in an urban African community*. Manchester: Manchester University Press.

Farmer, Paul. 1992. *AIDS and accusation: Haiti and the geography of blame*. Berkeley: University of California Press.

Fine, Gary Alan. 1988. Dying for a laugh: negotiating risk and creating personas in the humor of mushroom collectors. *Western Folklore* 47(Jul.): 177–194.

Fine, Gary Alan. 1992. *Manufacturing tales: Sex and money in contemporary legends*. Knoxville: University of Tennessee Press.

Finnegan, Ruth. 1970. Prose narratives I, problems and theories. *Oral literature in Africa*. London: Clarendon. pp. 315–334.

Foucault, Michel. 1978. *The history of sexuality, Vol. I: An Introduction*. Trans. Robert Hurley. New York": Pantheon.

Freud, Sigmund. 1950. *The interpretation of dreams*. New York: Random House, Inc.

Freud, Sigmund. 1960 [1909]. *Jokes and their relationship to the unconscious.* Trans. James Strachey. New York: Norton.

Fricke, Tom, et al. 1993. Marriage, social inequality, and women's contact with their natal families in alliance societies: two Tamang examples. *American Anthropologist, New Series* 95(Jun.): 395–419.

Friedson, Steven. 1996. *Dancing prophets: musical experience in Tumbuka healing.* Chicago: University of Chicago Press.

Geschiere, Peter. 1997. *The modernity of witchcraft: politics and the occult in post-colonial Africa.* Charlottesville: University of Virginia Press.

Gilman, Sander. 1988. *Disease and representation: images of illness from madness to AIDS.* Ithaca, NY: Cornell University Press.

Gluckman, Max. 1963. Gossip and scandal. *Current Anthropology* 4(3): 307–316.

Goffman, Ervin. 1974. *Frame analysis.* New York: Harper & Row.

Goldstein, Diane. 2004. *Once upon a virus: AIDS legends and vernacular risk perception.* Logan, Utah: Logan State University Press.

Gould, P. 1993. *The slow plague.* Oxford: Blackwell Publishers.

Griffiths, Anne.1997. *In the shadow of marriage: Gender and justice in an African community.* Chicago: University of Chicago Press

Hakansson, Thomas. 1994. The detachability of women: gender and kinship in processes of socioeconomic change among the Gusii of Kenya. *American Ethnologist* 21(Aug.): 516–538.

Harries, Anthony, et al. 2006. Scaling up antiretroviral treatment in resource-poor settings. *The Lancet* 367(Jun.): 1870–1872. www.thelancet.com

Harrison, Abigail and Elizabeth Montgomery. 2001. Life histories, reproductive histories: rural South African women's narratives of fertility, reproductive health and illness. *Journal of Southern African Studies, Special Issue on Fertility in Southern Africa* 27 (Jun.):311–328.

Hawthorne, Peter. 1999. An epidemic of rapes. *Time Magazine.* http://www.time.com/time/magazine/article/0,9171,992396–2,00.html.

Heise, Lori L. and Christopher Elias. 1995. Transforming AIDS prevention to meet women's needs: a focus on developing countries. *Social Science & Medicine* 40(7): 931–943.

HIV and AIDS Monitoring and Evaluation Report 2008–2009: UNGASS Country Progress Report.

Hufford, David. 1982. *The terror that comes in the night: an experience-centered study of supernatural assault traditions.* Philadelphia: University of Pennsylvania.

Hufford, David. 1995. Beings without bodies: an experience-centered theory of the belief in spirits. In *Out of the Ordinary: Folklore and the Supernatural.* ed. Barbara Walker, 11–45. Logan: University of Utah Press.

Hufford, David. 1996. Authority, knowledge, and substituted judgment. *Alternative therapies* 2(Nov): 92–94.

Hunt, C. W. 1989. Migrant labour and sexually transmitted diseases: AIDS in Africa. *Journal of. Health and Social Behavior* 30(4): 353–373.

Hunter, Mark. 2010. *Love in the time of AIDS: inequality, gender, and rights in South Africa*. Bloomington, IN: Indiana University Press.

Issiaka, S. et al. 2001. Living with HIV: women's experience in Burkina Faso, West Africa. *AIDS Care* 13(1): 123–128.

Jewkes, Rachel, et al. 2002. The virgin cleansing myth: cases of child rape are not exotic. *The Lancet* 359: 711.

Kachapila, Hendrina. 2006. The revival of *nyau* and changing gender relations in early colonial central Malawi. *Journal of Religion in Africa* 36(3–4): 319–345.

Kaler, Amy. 2001. "Many divorces and many spinsters": marriage as an invented tradition in southern Malawi, 1946–1999. *Journal of Family History* 26(Oct.): 529–556.

Kaler, Amy. 2003.My girlfriends could fill a yanu-yanu bus": Rural Malawian men's claims about their own serostatus. *Demographic Research*. September 19. www.demographic-research.org.

Kaler, Amy. 2004. AIDS-talk in everyday life: the presence of HIV/AIDS in men's informal conversation in Southern Malawi. *Social Science & Medicine* 59 (2004): 285–297.

Kaler, Amy. 2006. "When they see money, they think it's life": money, modernity and morality in two sites in rural Malawi. *Journal of Southern African Studies* 32(Jun.): 335–349.

Kandiyoti, Deniz. 1988. Bargaining with patriarchy. *Gender and Society* 2(Sept.): 274–290.

Kapferer, Bruce. 1972. *Strategy and transaction in an African factory: African workers and Indian management in a Zambian town*. Manchester: Manchester University Press.

Kapferer, Jean-Noel. 1990. *Rumors: uses, interpretations, and images*. New Brunswick, NJ: Transaction Publishers.

Kerr, Rachel, et al. 2008. "We grandmothers know plenty": breastfeeding, complementary feeding and the multifaceted role of grandmothers in Malawi. *Social Science & Medicine* 66: 1095–1105.

Kasenga, Fyson. 2010. Making it happen: prevention of mother to child transmission of HIV in rural Malawi. *Global Health Action* 3.

Kaspin, Deborah. 1995. The politics of ethnicity in Malawi's democratic transition. *Journal of Modern African Studies* 33(Dec,): 595–620.

Kerr, Rachel. 2005a. Food security in northern Malawi: gender, kinship relations and entitlements in historical context. *Journal of Southern African Studies* 31(1): 53–74.

Kerr, Rachel. 2005b. Informal labor and social relations in Northern Malawi: the theoretical challenges and implications of Ganyu labor for food security. *Rural Sociology* 70(2):167–187.

Kerr, Rachel, et al. 2008. "We grandmothers know plenty": breastfeeding, complementary feeding and the multifaceted role of grandmothers in Malawi. *Social Science & Medicine* 66: 1095–1105.

Kishindo, Pascal 1995. Sexual behaviour in the face of risk: the case of bar girls in Malawi's major cities. *Health Transition Review* 7(Suppl.): 153–160.

Kishindo, Pascal 2002 "Flogging" a dead cow?: The revivak of Malawin Chingoni. *Nordic Journal of African Studies* 11(2): 206–223.

Kligman, Gail. 1984. The rites of women: oral poetry, ideology, and the socialization of peasant women in contemporary Romania. *The Journal of American Folklore* 97 (Apr.–Jun.): 167–188.

Kuper, Hilda. 1958. Kinship among the Swazi. In *African Systems of Kinship and Marriage*. eds. A. R. Radcliffe-Brown and Daryll Forde. London: Oxford University Press.

Lane, T. 2004. In South Africa, wives' HIV prevention beliefs affect condom use with spouse. *International Family Planning Perspectives* 30(Sept.): 150–151.

Lawless, Sonia. 1996. Dirty, diseased and undeserving: the positioning of HIV positive women. *Social Science and Medicine* 43(9): 1371–1377.

Lesch, Elmien and Lou-Marie Kruger. 2005. Mothers, daughters and sexual agency in one low-income South African community. *Social Science & Medicine* 61: 1072–1082.

Libamba, Edwin, et al. 2007. Malawi's contribution to "3 by 5": achievements and challengers. *Bulletin of the World Health Organization*. 85(2).

Lloyd, Peter. 1968. Divorce among the Yuroba. *American Anthropologist, New Series* 70: 67–81.

Long, Norman. 1968. *Social change and the individual: a study of the social and religious responses to innovation in a Zambian rural community*. Manchester: Manchester University Press.

Luginaah, Isaac, et al. 2005. Challenges of a pandemic: HIV/AIDS-related problems affecting Kenyan widows. *Social Science & Medicine* 60: 1219–1228.Luke, Nancy. 2002a. The cultural significance of widowhood: widow inheritance and the position of Luo widows in the Kenya census. Paper presented at the Virtual Conference on African Households, Population Studies Center, University of Pennsylvania.

Luke, Nancy. 2002b. Widows and "professional inheritors": understanding AIDS risk perceptions in Kenya. Paper presented at the annual meetings of the Population Association of America, Atlanta.

Lwanda, John. 2005. *Politics, culture and medicine in Malawi*. Zomba, Malawi: Kachere Series.

Lloyd, Peter. 1968. Divorce among the Yuroba. *American Anthropologist, New Series* 70: 67–81.

Mair, L. P. 1953. African marriage and social change: southern Africa. In *Survey of African marriage and family life*. ed. Arthur Phillips.

Malawi Demographic Health Survey (MDHS) 2010. Published Sept. 2011 by Malawi's National Statistical Office. Zomba, Malawi.

Malungo, J. R. S. 2001. Sexual cleansing (*kusalazya*) and levirate marriage (*kunjilila mung'anda*) in the era of AIDS: changes in perceptions and practices in Zambia. *Social Science & Medicine* 53: 371–382.

Maman, S., et al. 2001. Women's barriers to HIV-1 testing and disclosure: challenges for HIV-1 voluntary counselling and testing. *AIDS Care* 13(5): 595–603.

Marwick, Max. 1965. *Sorcery in its social setting: a study of northern Rhodesian Cewa*. Manchester: Manchester University Press.

Mbilizi, Margaret. 1997. Gender socialization in education: accommodation and resistance by girls in Malawi schools. Indiana University, Ph.D. Dissertation.

McGrath, Janet W., et al. 1992. Cultural determinants of sexual risk behavior for AIDS among Baganda women. *Medical Anthropology Quarterly, New Series* 5(Jun.): 153–161.

Merry, Sally Engle. 1984. Rethinking gossip and scandal. In *Toward a General Theory of Social Control*, ed. Donald Black. 277–301. New York: Academic Press.

Mhalu, F., et al. 1991. A cross-sectional study of a program for HIV infection among public house workers. *Journal of Acquired Immune Deficiency Syndrome and Human Retrovirology* 4: 290–296.

Mitchell, Clyde. 1951. The Yao village of southern Nyasaland. In *Seven Tribes of Central Africa*, ed. Elizabeth Colson and Max Gluckman. 292–351.Manchester: Manchester University Press.

Mitchell, Clyde. 1956. *The Yao village: a* study *in the social structure of a Nyasaland tribe*. Manchester: Manchester University Press.

Morfit, Simon. 2011. "AIDS is money": how donor preferences reconfigure local realities. *World Development* 39: 64–76.

Morris, Brian. 1996. Chewa conceptions of disease. *Chewa Medical Botany: A study of herbalism in southern Malawi*. Hamburg: International African Institute.

Morris, Brian. 2000. *Animals and ancestors: an ethnography*. New York: Berg Publishers.

Morris, Brian. 2004. *Insects and human life*. Oxford: Berg.

Mutongi, Kenda. 1999. "Worries of the heart": widowed mothers, daughters and masculinities in Maragoli, Western Kenya, 1940–60. *The Journal of African History* 40(1): 67–86.

Muturi, Nancy and Samuel Mwangi. 2011. Older adults' perspectives on HIV/AIDS strategies for rural Kenya. *Health Communication* 26(8): 712–723.

National Statistical Office (NSO) [Malawi] and ORC Macro. 2005. Malawi demographic and health survey 2004. Calverton, Maryland: NSO and ORC Macro.

National Statistical Office (NSO) and ICF Macro. 2011. Malawi demographic and health survey 2010. Zomba, Malawi, and Calverton, Maryland, USA: NSO and ICF Macro.

Ngubane, Harriet. 1987. The consequences for women of marriage payments in a society with patrilineal descent. In *Transformations of African Marriage*, eds. David Parkin and David Nyamwaya. 173–182. Manchester: Manchester University Press.

Niraula, Bhanu and Philip Morgan. 1996. Marriage formation, post-marital contact with natal kin and autonomy of women: evidence from two Nepali settings. *Population Studies* 50: 35–50.

Ntozi, James P. M. 1997. Widowhood, remarriage and migration during the HIV/AIDS epidemic in Uganda. *Health Transition Review* 7(Suppl.): 125–144.

Obrdlik, Antonin. 1942. "Gallows humor"-a sociological phenomenon. *The American Journal of Sociology* 47: 709–716.

Okeyo, T. M. and Allen, A. K. 1994. Influence of widow inheritance on the epidemiology of AIDS in Africa. *African Journal of Medical Practice* I(1): 20–25.

Paine, Robert. 1967. What is gossip about? An alternative hypothesis. *Man, New Series* 2: 278–285.

Palella, Frank, et al. 1998. Declining morbidity and mortality among patient with advanced human immunodeficiency virus infection. *The New England Journal of Medicine* 338: 853–860.

Parker, R. G. 1987. Acquired immunodeficiency syndrome in urban Brazil. *Medical Anthropology Quarterly, New Series* 1(Jun.): 155–75.

Pass, Steven (ed.). 2004. *Chichewa-Chiyanja English Dictionary.* Kachere Series.

Peters, P. E., Kambewa, D., and P. A. Walker. 2010. Contestations over "tradition" and "culture" in a time of AIDS. *Medical Anthropology* 29(3): 278–302.

Peters, P. E., Kambewa, D., and P. A. Walker. 2008. The Effects of increasing rates of HIV/AIDS-related illness and death on rural families in Zomba District, Malawi: a longitudinal study. Report funded and coordinated by International Food Policy Research Institute and the Regional Network on AIDS Livelihoods and Food Security.

Phiri, Kings. 1983. Some changes in the matrilineal family system among the Chewa of Malawi since the nineteenth century. *Journal of African History* 24: 257–274.

Posner, Daniel. 2004. The political salience of cultural difference: why Chewas and Tumbukas are allies in Zambia and adversaries in Malawi. *American Political Science Review* 98(4): 529–545.

Poulin, Michelle. 2007. The sexual and social relations of youth in rural Malawi: strategies for AIDS prevention. PhD Dissertation, Boston University.

Power, Joey. 1995. "Eating the property": gender roles and economic change in urban Malawi, Blantyre-Limbe 1907–1953. *Journal of African Studies* 29(1):79–107.

Raybeck, Douglas. 1988. Anthropology and labeling theory: a constructive critique. *Ethos* 16(4): 371–397.

Reniers, Georges. 2003. Divorce and remarriage in rural Malawi. *Demographic Research,* Special Collection 1, Article 6. http://www.demographic-research.org.

Reniers, Georges. 2005. Marital strategies for managing the risk of HIV infection in rural Malawi. Presented at the Annual Population Association of America meeting, Philadelphia.

Reniers, Georges. 2006. HIV/AIDS surveillance and behavioral change in populations affected by the AIDS epidemic: four essays. PhD Dissertation, University of Pennsylvania.

Ribohn, Ulrika. 2002. "Human Rights and the multiparty system have swallowed our traditions": cConceiving women and culture in the new Malawi. In *A Democracy of Chameleons: Politics and Culture in the New Malawi,* ed. Harri Englund. 166–177. Blantyre: CLAIM/MABUKU.

Richards, Audrey. 1950. Some types of family structure amongst the Central Bantu. In *African Systems of Kinship and Marriage,* ed. A.R. Radcliffe-Brown and Daryll Forde. 207–251. London: Oxford University Press.

Roberts, John. 1964. The self-management of cultures. In *Explorations of Cultural Anthropology: Essays in honor of George Peter Murdock,* ed. Ward H. Goodenough. 433–454. New York: McGraw-Hill.

Robins, Steven. 2006. From "Rights" to "Ritual": AIDS activism in South Africa. *American Anthropologist* 108(2): 312–323.

Rödlach, Alexander. 2006. *Witches, westerners, and HIV: AIDS & cultures of blame in Africa.* Walnut Creek, CA: Left Coast Press Inc.

Rosenberg, Charles. 1987. *The cholera years.* Chicago: University of Chicago Press.

Rosenthal, Elisabeth. 2006. Traditional ways spread AIDS in Africa, experts say. *New York Times.* Nov. 21.

S. 1885. Popular poetry of the Esthonians. *The Folk-Lore Journal* 3(2):156–169.

Sabatier, Renée. 1988. *Blaming others: prejudice, race, and worldwide AIDS.* Washington: Panos Institute.

Sanders, Todd. 2003. Invisible hands and visible goods: revealed and concealed economies in millennial Tanzania. In *Transparency and Conspiracy: Ethnographers of Suspicion in the New World Order,* ed. Harry West and Todd Sanders. 148–174. Durham: Duke University Press.

Saur, Maria, et al. 2000. *Nkhanza: listening to peoples voices.* Zomba, Malawi: Kachere Series.

Schatz, Enid. 2002. Numbers and narratives: making sense of gender and context in rural Malawi. PhD dissertation, University of Pennsylvania.

Schmidt, Elizabeth. 1992. *Peasants, traders, and wives: Shona women in the history of Zimbabwe, 1870–1939.* London: Heinemann.

Schoepf, Brooke. 1988. Women, AIDS, and economic crisis in central Africa. *Canadian Journal of African Studies* 22(3): 625–644.

Schoepf, Brooke. 2001. International AIDS research in anthropology: taking a critical perspective on the crisis. *Annual Review of Anthropology* 30: 335–361.

Schoffeleers, Matthew. 1999. The AIDS pandemic, the prophet Billy Chisupe, and the democratization process in Malawi. *Journal of Religion in Africa* 29(Fasc. 4): 406–441.

Seeley, Janet, et al. 1994. Socioeconomic Status, gender, and risk of HIV-1 Infection in a rural community in South West Uganda. *Medical Anthropology Quarterly, New Series*. 8: 78–89.

Setel, Philip. 1999. Population, men, and movement: (M)oral demographies of desire and risk. In *A plague of paradoxes: AIDS, culture, and demography in Northern Tanzania*, 51–88. Chicago: University of Chicago.

Shevory, Thomas. 2004. *Notorious H.I.V.: the media spectacle of Nushawn Williams*. Minneapolis, MN: University of Minnesota Press.

Shibutani, Tamotsu. 1966. *Improvised news: a sociological study of rumor.* Indianapolis: Bobbs-Merrill.

Sinding, Steven. 2005. Does "CNN" (Condoms, Needles and Negotiation) work better than 'ABC' (Abstinence, Being Faithful and Condom Use) in attacking the AIDS Epidemic? *International Family Planning Perspectives* 31: 38–40.

Smith, Kirsten. 2003. Why are they worried?: Concern about HIV/AIDS in rural Malawi. *Demographic Research. Special Collection* 1(9).

Smith, Kirsten and Susan Watkins. 2005. Perceptions of risk and strategies for prevention: responses to HIV/AIDS in rural Malawi. *Social Science & Medicine* 60: 649–660.

Stadler, Jonathan. 2003. Rumor, gossip and blame: implications for HIV/AIDS prevention in the South African lowveld. *AIDS Education and Prevention* 15(4): 357–368.

Stewart, Charles. 2002. Erotic dreams and nightmares from antiquity to present. *The Journal of the Royal Anthropological Institute* 8(2): 279–309.

Stewart, Pamela and Andrew Strathern. 2004. *Witchcraft, sorcery, rumors, and gossip*. Cambridge: Cambridge University Press.

Swidler, Ann. 2006. Syncretism and subversion in AIDS governance: how locals cope with global demands. *International Affairs* 82(2): 269–284.

Swidler, Ann and Susan Watkins. 2005. Hearsay ethnography. Paper presented at the Annual Meeting of the Population Association of America, Philadelphia.

Takane, Tsutomu. 2006. Risky business: smallholder tobacco production and rural livelihoods in Malawi. In *Current issues of rural development in Malawi*. 133–174. Chiba, Japan: Institute of Developing Economies.

Treichler, Paula. 1999. *How to have theory in an epidemic*. Durham: Duke University Press.

Turner, Patricia. 1993. *I heard it through the grapevine: rumor in African-American culture*. Berkeley: University of California Press.

Turner, Victor. 1996 [1957]. *Schism and continuity in African society: a study of Ndembu village Life*. Oxford: Berg.

Turner, W. (compiler) 1996 [1952] *chiTumbuka/chiTonga—English and English—Tumbuka/Tonga Dictionary*. Blantyre, Malawi: Central Africana Limited.

Ulin, P. R. 1992. African women and AIDS: negotiating behavioral change. *Social Science & Medicine* 34(1): 63–73.

UN World Food Program 2010 Rural Malawi Comprehensive Security and Vulnerability Analysis.

Vail, Leroy and Landeg White. 1989. Tribalism in the political history of Malawi. In *The creation of tribalism in southern Africa*, ed. Leroy Vail. 151–92. Berkeley and Los Angeles: University of California Press.

van Breugel, J. W. M. 2001 *Chewa traditional religion*. Zomba, Malawi: Kachere Series.

van Velsen, J. 1967. The extended-case method and situational analysis. In *The craft of social anthropology*, ed. A. L. Epstein. 129–149. London: Tavistock.

Waldby, C. 1996. *AIDS and the body politic*. London: Routledge Press.

Walden, Vivien, et al. 1999. Measuring the impact of a behaviour change intervention for commercial sex workers and their potential clients in Malawi. *Health Education Research* 14(4): 545–554.

Warner, Faith. 2007. Social support and distress among Q'eqchi' refugee women in Maya Tecún, Mexico. *Medical Anthropology Quarterly* 21(Jun.):193–217.

Watkins, Susan. 2004. Navigating the AIDS epidemic in Rural Malawi. *Population and Development Review* 30 (Dec.): 673–705.

West, Harry and Tracy Luedke. 2006. Healing divides: therapeutic border work in southeast Asia. In *Borders and Healers: Brokering Therapeutic Resources in Southeast Africa*. 1–20. Bloomington and Indianapolis: Indiana University Press.

White, Landeg. 1987. *Magomero: portrait of an African village*. Cambridge: Cambridge University Press.

White, Luise. 2000. *Speaking with vampires: rumor and history in colonial Africa*. Berkeley: University of California Press.

Whyte, Susan Reynolds. 1997. *Questioning misfortune: the pragmatics of uncertainty in eastern Uganda*. Cambridge, UK: Cambridge University Press.

Wilson, Anika. 2008. "There is no secret under the sun": Rumors, AIDS beliefs, and prevention strategies of wives in Malawi. PhD Dissertation, University of Pennsylvania.

Wilson, Anika. 2012. Of love potions and witch baskets: domesticity, mobility, and occult rumors in Malawi. *Western Folklore* 71:2 (Spring 2012) :149–173.

WLSA (Women and Law in Southern Africa Research Trust). 2000. *In search of justice: women and the administration of justice in Malaŵi*. Dzuka Publishing Company Limited.

WLSA (Women and Law in Southern Africa Research and Educational Trust). 2009. Malawi CEDAW Shadow Report.

Yamba, C. Bawa. 1997. Cosmologies in turmoil: witchfinding and AIDS in Chiawa, Zambia. *Journal of the International African Institute* 67(1997): 200–223.

Young, T. Cullen, 1931. *Notes on the customs and folklore of the Tumbuka-Kamanga Peoples*. Livingstonia: The Mission Press.

Zuberi, Tukufu and Amson Sibanda. 2004. How do migrants fare in a post-apartheid South African labor market? *International Migration Review* 38(4): 1462–1491.

Zulu, Eliya. 2001. Ethnic variations in observance and rationale for postpartum sexual abstinence in Malawi. *Demography* 38(Nov): 467–479.

INDEX

Printed and bound by CPI Group (UK) Ltd, Croydon, CR0 4YY